# OPTIMAL FITNESS THROUGH RECREATIONAL SPORTS

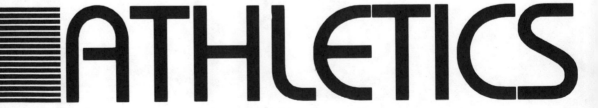

ATHLETICS

# Kenneth Forsythe, M.D., and Neil Feineman

A Fireside Book
Published by Simon & Schuster, Inc.
New York

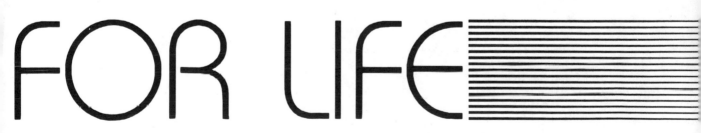

FOR LIFE

Simon and Schuster/Fireside Books
Published by Simon & Schuster, Inc.
Simon & Schuster Building
Rockefeller Center
1230 Avenue of the Americas
New York, New York 10020
All photographs in this book are copyright © Roger Allyn Lee
SIMON AND SCHUSTER, FIRESIDE and colophons are registered
trademarks of Simon & Schuster, Inc.
Designed by Karolina Harris
Manufactured in the United States of America
10 9 8 7 6 5 4 3 2 1
10 9 8 7 6 5 4 3 2 1 pbk.
Library of Congress Cataloging in Publication Data
Forsythe, Kenneth.
    Athletics for life.

    "A Simon and Schuster/Fireside Book."
    Bibliography: p.
    1. Physical education and training.    2. Sports.    3. Physical fit-
ness. 4. Aerobic exercises.
I. Feineman, Neil.    II. Title.
GV711.5.F67   1985      613.7'1    85-18247
ISBN: 0-671-53123-9
ISBN: 0-671-61777-X pbk.

# TO OUR PARENTS

WE would like to thank the people who made this book possible, including our agents, Maureen and Eric Lasher; our editor, Donald Hutter; Catherine Shaw, Katherine Vaz, and Heidi Yorkshire; the staff at ALTA Institute; Doug Emery; Dr. Jay Kenney, Ph.D.; Roger Lee; John and Francis Slouber, of the Royal Gorge Ski Resort; and Per Astrand, for his inspiration.

# Acknowledgments

As CHAIRMAN of the President's Council on Physical Fitness, one of my most rewarding experiences has been to watch the continued commitment more Americans are making to physical fitness. In the past several years, adults, especially women, in this country have made great strides toward a more healthful level of fitness. And our young athletes have never been in better shape. It wasn't so long ago that Americans had lost their enthusiasm for exercise and were slipping into a sedentary and unhealthful life-style.

Now, the attitude toward physical activity has changed dramatically. In the last four and one-half years, the President's Council has made great strides in making millions of Americans aware of the importance of good exercise and nutrition habits. When I was in school, we learned very little about nutrition, flexibility, or exercise. We did many things that were wrong, such as deep knee bends, straight-leg sit-ups, and duck waddles. Luckily, today's active adults have the correct information and our children have it from the start.

Despite this information, youth fitness still remains my top priority. Many kids who are not going out for sports are in poor shape; they are not strong, have no cardiovascular fitness, and have a high percentage of body fat.

Also, many adults are still not exercising. While fitness has become a priority for so many of us, 100 million adults have not yet realized the importance of regular physical activity, denying themselves the joys of health. This hurts the country by leading to reduced productivity, increased absence on the job, unnecessary illness, and even premature mortality.

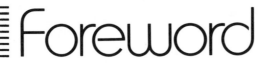 Foreword

Reaching these people is not easy. When I was coaching, I had no problem finding ways to motivate my players to meet the demands of my program. But now, faced with the task of motivating 200 million Americans, I find the job more challenging. Direct personal contact with everyone, as well as the luxury of seeing day-to-day results, is impossible.

Even with these practical limitations, the Council remains extremely committed to changing the health of our nation. There are many projects in the country aimed at increasing fitness awareness. An example is the U.S. Fitness Academy, possibly to be situated in Southern California and scheduled to open in 1988. It will be a clearinghouse for information on diet, health, nutrition, sports medicine, sports research, and fitness. It will train qualified fitness instructors and will offer short-term seminars on a variety of health- and fitness-related concerns to all Americans.

To win the battle for fitness, we also need programs like *Athletics for Life*. What strikes me most about this excellent, complete new approach to exercise is its integration of a sound mental approach to fitness with a physically challenging and enjoyable format. By using it, both the young and old can take advantage of solo and team sports and enjoy the benefits a healthy mind and body can bring.

As the President's Council's brochure states: "The responsibility for action rests with parents, school administrators, teachers, coaches, recreation supervisors, civic and business leaders, and other individuals. In other words, it's up to you. We hope you'll do your part." With this book, that effort should be much easier and more productive. It is a pleasure to recommend *Athletics for Life*.

—George Allen

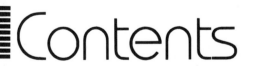 Contents

FITNESS books have become almost as numerous as the number of people exercising. One couldn't be blamed for wondering why there should be another. But the fitness revolution has come to a crossroads and is in danger of taking the wrong path.

Millions of Americans already are suffering from unnecessary exercise-induced injuries. Millions more participate in exercise programs that are supposed to produce weight loss but don't. Recreational sports that could provide cardiopulmonary benefits aren't doing so. Exercise burnout from overly stressful programs is becoming epidemic. And thousands of people who have been exercising for years are thirsting for improvement but can't get better at their sport.

To understand why, you must go back twenty years, to the dark ages of American fitness. Back then, smoking was chic. Most people had diets high in fat and considered them healthful. Exercise was something you did in high school, if then, and "aerobics" was a physiological term that the lay public had not yet heard.

Then, in the mid-'60s, a maverick doctor, Ken Cooper, explained aerobics in his now world-famous book of the same name. He argued that sustained regular exercise of a certain intensity could prevent cardiovascular disease. Now the idea seems commonplace, but then it was radical and actively derided by much of the medical community. Despite their skepticism, however, the public was thirsty for information about fitness and, more importantly, ready to work out.

Over the next few years, joggers became a common sight along America's roadways. Thousands of others worked out in their homes with programs like the Canadian Air Force exercises, or joined tennis or racquetball clubs. More bicycles were sold than cars; middle-class America learned how to ski; and aerobic dance became a national mania.

With notable exceptions such as Dr. Cooper himself, the medical community did little to lead the fitness revolution. As a result, the movement is now led by movie stars and lay entrepreneurs who, though devoted and

# Fitness: The Third Wave 1

well-intentioned exponents of the active life-style, are often misinformed. Their programs are usually ineffective in terms of weight control and the prevention of cardiopulmonary disease, cause an unnecessarily high incidence of sports-related injuries, and fail to bring about improved levels of performance.

Losing weight is perhaps the most popular reason for beginning an exercise program. Yet countless people have exercised for months or years without losing weight, and now mistakenly have abandoned exercise in discouragement. Of course diet and psychological issues play a role in weight loss, yet exercise that is performed correctly holds the key to long-term weight control.

Cardiopulmonary health is also a vitally important goal of any fitness program. That is why millions of Americans are regularly engaged in aerobics, swimming, cycling, and racquet sports, which they think provide them with optimal cardiopulmonary health. In reality, however, their fitness level is not much different from that of a sedentary adult of the same age. Despite their efforts, they are not as healthy as they think.

Misinformed exercise programs are also producing injuries at an alarming rate. Sixty percent of the joggers and 65 percent of the aerobic dancers in this country have suffered an exercise-induced injury. Unfortunately, too many people conclude that it is the exercise that is to blame, not their lack of knowledge as to how to safely perform the activity.

Finally, for better or worse, most Americans are concerned about their performance. Millions of us have jogged, skied, played tennis, and cycled for years without improving at the activity. Most of us eventually become frustrated by these plateaus. Because the approach to training for peak performance has never been explained to those involved in recreational sports, attempts to improve are usually self-directed and misguided, and result only in increased boredom, burnout, or worse, injuries. This is lamentable, because performance gains are possible for almost anyone.

To further convince you of the gravity of the situation, we will examine some of the common exercise myths. Legacies of years of misconception and misinformation, they are undermining the success of the fitness revolution and undoing many of the inroads already made.

# The Myths of Fitness

## Myth one: I look fit, so I don't have to exercise

Almost no one is envied more than the person who eats whatever he wants without gaining weight. Jim, a thirty-two-year-old lawyer who could do that, bragged that he didn't watch his diet but still had not gained a pound since college. He never exercised, in part because his work left him too tired to do anything more than collapse when he got home.

He came to me for a physical, and was surprised that the procedure involved more than taking his blood pressure and weight and doing some cursory blood work. In one of our tests, for example, I measured his body composition, or ratio of fat to lean body mass, with a pair of calipers. This is a far more vital statistic than weight, because it measures exactly how much of your body is fat and how much is lean body tissue. If you weighed one hundred sixty pounds and had only a lean, ten-percent body fat, for instance, about only sixteen pounds of your weight would be fat. Jim weighed one hundred sixty pounds but had a body composition of twenty-five-percent body fat. He thus had to carry around forty pounds of fat.

A certain amount of fat is necessary—for insulating the body, maintaining normal core temperature, storing energy, and, to a small extent, metabolizing certain hormones. Excess amounts, however, are undesirable. We are only now uncovering the direct relationship between obesity and many common medical problems, but the indirect and probably causal relationship between obesity and high blood pressure, musculoskeletal problems, and cardiovascular disease is well established.

At first, Jim could not believe that he was statistically obese, because he didn't look fat. Obesity, however, is not simply a case of round and roly lumps and bumps over the belt, but an unhealthfully large percentage of body fat relative to lean body tissue, which is made up primarily of muscle and bones.

Since regular exercise is by far the most effective way of lowering the percentage of fat, Jim agreed to give it a try. He wanted an activity that got him outdoors and away from his office, so he decided to take up cycling. Four times a week he rode the bicycle at an energizing but not exhausting pace for thirty to forty-five minutes.

Cycling is a lower-body sport, which means it primarily involves the legs.

To balance that and develop his shoulders and arms, Jim also began swimming, an excellent upper-body workout, several times a week. Within a few months, his percentage of body fat had been reduced to the healthy range. Even though he had never felt or looked unhealthy, he was amazed at how much better he felt—and how much more toned he looked—after a few months of mild but regular exercise.

### Myth two: I'm active, so I don't have to exercise

When she came to see me, Jane, who is fifty-two years old, considered herself quite knowledgeable about health matters. She ate a balanced diet and was within the height/weight guidelines of the standard Metropolitan Life Insurance tables. She did not exercise regularly because she thought she was active enough, what with walking up and down the stairs of her family's three-story house all day, doing all of her own housework, and playing a weekly game of tennis. She too came to me for a physical thinking that nothing was really wrong with her.

She took the exercise treadmill test, in which levels of aerobic fitness are monitored—this is the best indication of how efficiently the heart and lungs are working. To her surprise, her score was that of a sedentary adult in her age group.

Like many tennis players, swimmers, and cyclists who assume that they are active enough to protect their hearts and lungs but get disappointing results on the treadmill, Jane questioned the accuracy of the test. But she soon realized that her activities were not elevating the heart rate or increasing the demand for oxygen in the muscles sufficiently to promote cardiopulmonary fitness. To do that, exercise must involve large groups of the body's muscle mass and be performed at a sufficiently high intensity in a continuous manner for at least twenty minutes.

To improve Jane's aerobic fitness, we devised a more vigorous and regular exercise program for her. At first, she briskly walked three miles every morning. Four weeks later she jogged one street and walked the next. By the end of another month, she slowly jogged the entire three miles. Before long, her aerobic capacity improved, reflecting a healthier cardiovascular system.

## Myth three: twenty minutes of exercise three times a week is all you need

Charles, a fifty-seven-year-old accountant, followed the advice of his cardiologist and jogged for twenty minutes three times a week. Despite this exercise, he couldn't seem to lose weight, was not sleeping well, and couldn't handle the stress of his job well. Exercise was supposed to help in these matters, so why, he wondered, wasn't he benefiting more from his program?

Three twenty-minute sessions weekly result in a more efficient cardiopulmonary system, he learned, but this is rarely sufficient to control weight or stress. To do that, exercise must be performed daily at a moderate intensity for thirty to sixty minutes.

Understandably, Charles resisted the idea of daily exercise. Simply finding the time to exercise every day at first seemed to add to, rather than reduce, the already considerable amount of stress in his life. Fortunately, I prevailed upon him to give the program a try.

Charles was already able to jog for twenty minutes, but he made some technical mistakes in his form that prematurely tired him. By reducing the length of his stride and keeping his heart rate at slightly lower levels than before, he soon was able to run for forty-five minutes without feeling exhausted. On alternate days he went to a YMCA near his office and swam laps. Within a month, he had lost eight pounds and was sleeping more soundly than he had in years. Originally skeptical, he now knew that daily, low-intensity exercise is a potent remedy for a stressful executive life-style.

## Myth four: the more you exercise, the better off you'll be

Joe, a twenty-five-year-old waiter whose hobby was running in amateur races, had no problem with the concept of daily exercise. He believed that "more is better," running three hours a day and more than one hundred miles a week. He won many of his races but was frequently plagued by minor injuries.

Joe came to me for treatment of a fatigue fracture in his lower leg, a painful result of his overly intense training program. The constant pounding had caused microscopic deformities in the shinbone, a painful condition commonly called a stress fracture. To recover, Joe had to avoid jogging and any other weight-bearing activity for three weeks. To maintain his cardiopulmonary fitness during this time, he rode a stationary bicycle for forty-five minutes a day at prescribed but varying intensities. At the end of the three weeks, he started running again, but for shorter distances and at varying intensities.

Two months later Joe ran his best marathon in two years. His fatigue fracture had been a blessing in disguise, because it forced him to curtail his self-destructive overtraining. Like many other athletes, he mistakenly believed that the more training he could cram in, the better he would get. Instead, overtraining had led only to poor performance and injury.

### Myth five: no pain, no gain

Lynn, a thirty-one-year-old nurse, was victimized by another popular version of overtraining, the "no pain, no gain" philosophy. She joined a health club two years ago and rapidly got caught up in the competitive atmosphere of the exercise class. The instructor barked to "go for the burn," or the painful sensation that overtired muscles emit, and Lynn dutifully obeyed.

She went to the health club five times a week, and worked to her maximum capacity each time. After a few months, she was fed up with being constantly exhausted. Because she always pushed herself to new levels, the classes never became easier. Then her Achilles tendons and knees started to ache. She decided that the physical and mental struggle wasn't worth it, and stopped exercising altogether.

Some time later she consulted me because she wanted to lose the weight she had gained in the interim, but she bridled when I mentioned exercise. Considering her arduous and unpleasant experience, exercise was an effort she did not want to undertake again.

Lynn was surprised but happy to learn, then, that the most effective exercise for weight loss is moderate in intensity, rather than strenuous or painful. As Lynn's case proves, strenuous exercise sessions tend to be shorter in duration and generally result in exercise burnout if performed day after day. Moderate exercise, on the other hand, is almost always perceived as pleasant. Longer workouts are tolerated, and the exercise program becomes much easier to stick to for extended periods of time.

Even more important, the body's primary source of fuel during moderate exercise is fatty acids, which are taken from the body's fat stores. In strenuous exercise, the body takes its fuel primarily from carbohydrates in the muscles. Exercise of moderate intensity burns more calories because it is performed longer and burns fat, which is what most people are trying to lose.

Encouraged, Lynn started the next day with a combination walking and jogging program, which she felt would be most convenient for her. She soon started losing weight, which boosted her confidence and her commitment. Within a month, she could jog for almost the entire exercise session. Within three months, she was also taking occasional exercise classes, and pacing herself through them so that they were fun and not torturous.

### Myth six: cutting calories is the best way to lose weight

Gary, a twenty-eight-year-old stockbroker, was self-conscious about his body and desperately wanted to lose thirty-five pounds. He had tried a variety of low-calorie diets, and usually lost ten or twelve pounds. But the weight always crept back on.

Gary was fighting a familiar losing battle. More than 90 percent of the people who lose weight by just dieting regain it within a year. We are still learning about the intricate mechanisms of weight control, but an important new theory backed by a considerable body of evidence helps explain why the failure rate is so high.

This theory suggests that there is a central mechanism in the brain called the apestat, which helps control metabolism and energy demands. Like a thermostat set at a certain temperature, the apestat sets the body's weight. If the weight level goes too high, the apestat adjusts the metabolism to return to the set weight. If the weight goes too low the apestat makes another adjustment and brings the weight back up.

The apestat obviously is not the only factor in weight control, or it would be impossible to gain or lose weight. But it may be a factor in determining the metabolic rate, and thus helps explain why the body rejects our attempts at rapid weight loss. We think it takes from eight to ten months to reset the apestat. Once it is reset, the apestat helps you stop overeating and keeps you at your new weight.

The long readjustment period at least in part explains why six hundred-to eight hundred-calorie-a-day diets don't work. Most people cannot adhere to such a restrictive diet for long. One doctor at the University of Southern California who is investigating obesity reports that many of his patients swore they stuck to their diets but couldn't lose weight. Finding it difficult to believe that someone could eat six hundred calories per day and not lose weight, he enrolled a group of them in an in-house program that monitored all of their activities for several weeks. Invariably, when strictly monitored and forced to keep to the diet, the patients lost weight. When outside the hospital, they apparently "forgot" about some of the calories they consumed.

Rather than try another unrealistic diet, Gary began jogging and cycling at an easy pace four times a week and lifting weights twice a week. The weights built lean muscle tissue, and the aerobic exercise burned calories and fat. He also made modest modifications in his diet, shifting from foods that were high in fat to those high in complex carbohydrates. Together these changes proved a potent combination, and allowed him to go from 32-percent body fat to 25-percent body fat and drop ten pounds in three months. Because the dietary changes were modest and the exercise pleasant, Gary enjoyed his new life-style. Without feeling deprived or resentful, he has maintained a twenty-five-pound weight loss for over a year.

## Myth seven: spot reduction is all most women need

Tracy, an aerobics teacher in her late twenties, came to me because she was suffering from debilitating hip pains. She often had to teach two advanced classes back to back, and had been lying down on a floor mat and leading each class in hundreds of leg lifts.

I examined her hip and leg, and found that she had a great deal of tenderness in her gluteus medius muscle, the muscle primarily responsible for raising the leg sideway during the exercise. I asked her why she had the class do the exercise, and she gave me the predictable answer: It was the best way to lose fat and firm up the hips.

Although widely believed, the concept of reducing fat in a particular part of the body is as nonsensical as it is harmful. In the first place, spot reduction is physiologically impossible. Women store fat in certain places—such as the breasts, abdomen, and thighs—and men in others—such as the abdomen and back. But these are just storage areas, and exercising the muscles underneath them will not burn the fat lying on top of the muscles. When fat is burned, it is burned from all over. By far the best way to do that is through aerobic exercise.

Spot-reduction exercises don't work because they don't use enough muscle mass to elevate the body's metabolism to fat-burning levels. In fact, while exercises that isolate specific muscles may be fine for body builders trying to develop bulges in every part of their bodies, they are less likely to benefit anyone else. The isolation usually succeeds only in fatiguing the muscle, leaving it more susceptible to strains, tears, and other injuries.

Tracy adjusted the structure of her class to include more full-body movements that used increased amounts of muscle groups in a full range of motion. The increased aerobic activity made the class more effective. Within a few weeks, the tenderness in her gluteus medius muscle was gone. Thanks to her revised workout, it has not returned.

### Myth eight: cellulite treatments work

Along similar lines, Jennifer, a thirty-eight-year-old legal secretary, asked me how she could get rid of her cellulite. She had spent considerable amounts of money on creams, lotions, and body wraps, and couldn't understand why they didn't work.

Even though it has spawned a multimillion-dollar industry, best-selling books, and legions of believers who swear they are afflicted with it, cellulite is only a word invented by a French cosmetologist who came to New York many years ago and reputedly became very wealthy selling people substances that supposedly removed it.

An elementary knowledge of the body's composition, however, explains why these creams and lotions can't work. Most of the body's fat rests just under the skin in what is called the subcutaneous layer. These adipose, or fat, cells are little, round, globule-like balls. Unlike muscle tissue, which is smooth, fat is lumpy. When present in sufficient number, these pea-shaped cells cause the dimpling of the skin referred to as cellulite.

Lotions and creams cannot burn up this fat. Neither can body wrapping, which may reduce girth in some people temporarily, because the fat cells are compressible. Like a pillow that only briefly holds the indentation of your head after a full night's sleep, the fat cells will regain their original shape in a short period of time.

To get rid of her cellulite, Jennifer had to give up her reliance on passive solutions and engage in daily aerobic exercise. She had always wanted to play tennis, so I devised a tennis program that was aerobic, challenging, and entertaining. Six months later, her "cellulite" and several percentage points of body fat were gone.

### Myth nine: stretch before you exercise

Peter, a twenty-four-year-old collegiate champion runner, had suffered from chronic pain in the back of his upper right thigh and buttocks for two-

and-one-half years. I watched him work out and noticed that as soon as he got to the track, he put his foot up on the wall and stretched his hamstrings. When I asked why he stretched, he looked surprised. Didn't everyone?

Like most of us, he had heard so much about the importance of stretching before you exercise that he thought it was an exercise basic. Unfortunately, however, the practice has no basis in fact. At normal resting temperature, the connective tissue in the muscles is relatively inelastic and prone to microscopic tears. Only when the blood supply to the muscles increases and warms the muscles does the tissue become more flexible.

To heal the muscle, I used a type of treatment involving electromagnetic fields. To solve the larger problem of preactivity stretching, which was the underlying cause of the pain, I told him to warm up by doing the activity at a very low level for ten minutes and to save the stretching for after the aerobic segment of the workout, when his tissues were warm and distensible. Now, one year later, he stretches *after* his workouts and has had no further problems.

While the specifics of each of these people's problems are different, they all shared the goals of improved health, appearance, and performance. Yet despite a uniformly high level of intelligence and in some cases extensive involvement in the exercise field, none knew how to establish a safe and scientifically sound exercise program that would satisfy these goals.

After seeing too many patients who were needlessly discouraged, unnecessarily hurt, or not improving, I became convinced that it was time to go beyond what was currently available and develop a scientifically valid, individualized, and realistic fitness program built around the most popular recreational sports. The result, *Athletics for Life*, is based on my experience as a competitive skier, tennis player, runner, cyclist, and triathlete, and as a sports medicine physician. By using the most current scientific research and the training secrets of the world's top athletes, the workouts place optimal fitness within everyone's reach.

## Safe Exercise

Especially in light of the increasing numbers of exercise casualties physicians around the country are seeing, my first concern was that the program must be safe. Unlike many programs, which can cause injury, *Athletics for Life* builds safety into its design because it is written from both a physician's and an athlete's point of view. It carefully details the hazards involved in each sport and explains how to avoid them. It also keeps the exercise sessions at a reasonable intensity and duration, thus preventing injuries resulting from overexertion or fatigue.

## Effective Exercise

The workouts in this book result in cardiopulmonary fitness. Although this may seem to you an assumption that goes without saying, many, if not most, fitness books do not adequately provide for even this basic goal of an exercise program. As popularly practiced, cycling, swimming, tennis, downhill skiing, raquetball, and aerobic dancing are often not done in ways that provide aerobic benefits, even though all are potentially great aerobic activities. *Athletics for Life* solves this problem by showing you how to adjust each sport so that it becomes aerobic.

But aerobic, or cardiopulmonary, concerns are only part of an optimal fitness program. Weight control, stress management, alleviation of back pain and other common musculoskeletal problems, and improving strength and athletic performances are also important concerns that a well-developed fitness program should deal with. Few, however, do.

Most weight-loss programs, for instance, have a failure rate of over 95 percent, which means that only five out of every one hundred people are able to maintain that weight loss for more than six months. *Athletics for Life* shows you how to achieve permanent weight loss because it emphasizes the gradual reduction of the percentage of body fat through minor dietary modifications and workouts of tolerable intensity. When you reach your healthful body composition, you will also arrive at your healthful weight, generally without having to count calories or make unrealistic dietary changes.

In addition to weight control, *Athletics for Life* shows you how to develop all the muscles in the body. People who participate in only one sport often develop imbalances, or areas of weakness, that can lead to injury. To call these previously unused muscles into play, *Athletics for Life* provides drills and supplemental exercises that strengthen and tone complementary muscles as well as the ones required by the particular sport. Not only is it more effective, but this kind of training also leads to a more sculptured-looking body, because all the muscle groups are strengthened.

## Enjoyable Workouts

Finally, to be successful the fitness program must be enjoyable. Unlike other programs, which force you to exercise within their repetitive and ultimately restrictive structures, *Athletics for Life* allows you to enjoy your program by centering on the six most popular participant sports in the country: running, bicycling, racquet sports, skiing, swimming, and aerobic dancing. It explains how you can improve your performance and make each one aerobically satisfying.

Then, if you wish, it integrates one or any number of sports that you enjoy into a comprehensive and challenging fitness program. For instance you may like to ski in the winter and play tennis in the spring, or divide your athletic efforts between running and swimming. *Athletics for Life* shows you how to coordinate changes like these into a consistent though varied training program.

## The Benefits of Cross-Training

*Athletics for Life* thus introduces you to cross-training, a recently popularized development in fitness. In cross-training, your performance in one sport benefits by your performance in another. Running, for example, requires significant cardiopulmonary power, but this power does not have to be gained from running. Cycling also develops cardiopulmonary power effectively, and it has the additional characteristic of being a nongravity, and subsequently less stressful, sport. Cross-training with cycling, then, is an ideal way to relieve the unrelenting pounding on the musculoskeletal system of daily running and still build cardiopulmonary power.

In addition to the safety factor, training regularly in several different sports helps you stay fresh in each. As an added advantage, you will develop a more balanced body through multisport training because you exercise all the muscle groups, rather than just the muscles used in one specific sport.

## STEP—The Specific Training Exercise Program

Participating in one sport, however, does not automatically result in improvements in another sport, because the first sport does not necessarily prepare the right muscles for the specific demands of the second one. An accomplished swimmer will have very good aerobic power, for instance, but that is no guarantee that he will run well. Swimming is primarily an upper-body sport and does little to prepare the legs for the stresses of running.

To train the muscles for the specific movements of particular sports, I have developed STEP. It is a group of specially devised exercises that prepare the muscles for a specific sport. Most recreational skiers, for example, cannot ski for at least the first few days without noticeable fatigue and pain. The *Athletics for Life* program, however, features several months of preseason ski drills that develop the muscles necessary for the sport and thus help the skier come to the slopes already prepared for the sport's demands.

## Training for Competition

Since maintaining fitness or performance levels is different from training for peak performance, maximum improvement, or competitive events, *Athletics for Life* includes two different training schedules. The first is the maintenance program, which is composed primarily of moderate-intensity workouts of long duration. You will use these workouts most of the year.

During the time that you want to peak, however, you should shift into the optional-training workouts, which are more demanding. They use a variety of training techniques, often performed at a higher intensity, for three months. By the end of that period, you will be at your most finely tuned. If desired, you can also adjust these training periods and achieve a more moderate rate of improvement, but with less all-out effort.

## Fitness: The Third Wave

*Athletics for Life*, then, results in optimal fitness because it controls your weight, improves your cardiopulmonary condition, tones both your upper and lower body muscles, reduces stress, and teaches you how to improve in the sport or sports of your choice. It is adaptable to your changing desires, interests, demands, situations, or environment, taking you beyond the many ill-defined notions surrounding aerobics to the next step—a life of fitness, health, and athletic achievement you thought was unattainable.

THERE is a great deal of talk these days about "aerobics," but few people, I have found, really know what the term means. Simply speaking, aerobics is any sustained exercise that forces the heart and lungs to pump a certain amount of oxygen into the muscles. This effort increases the efficiency of the cardiopulmonary system and of the metabolism of the muscles themselves.

As you know from the first chapter, not all exercise is sufficiently intense to be aerobic. For it to be aerobic, three conditions must be met. First, during the exercise the heart must beat at 65 percent or more of its maximal rate. (To find out your maximum heart rate, or how fast your heart can beat at its maximal effort, subtract 65 percent of your age from 210. See Target Heart Rate chart, Appendix 1.)

Sixty-five percent of your maximum heart rate, the lowest point at which you begin to derive aerobic benefits from exercise, is called the aerobic threshold. Some types of exercise never get you to this threshold. Doing bicep curls all day, for example, would provide no aerobic benefit because this exercise does not use enough muscle mass. Other sports, such as swimming, use large muscle masses but still may not push you into the aerobic threshold. Because water buoys the body, many swimmers are not working as intensely as they think. To avoid making the same mistake, check your heart rate as you exercise.

It is possible to increase the heart rate by means other than exercise. Sitting in a sauna or experiencing an adrenalin-producing fright may elevate the heart rate, but for aerobic benefits to be derived, the source of the increase must be from the work of the body's muscles. Thus, the second criterion is that the exercise involve a significant portion of the body's muscles.

Finally, research has shown that the beneficial changes to the heart, such as improved vascularity (more capillaries) and increased strength (or stroke volume), occur only when exercise of a certain minimal intensity has been sustained for fifteen minutes. A shorter session will not generate any of the

# 2 The Basics of Aerobics

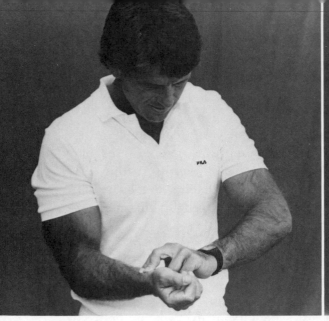
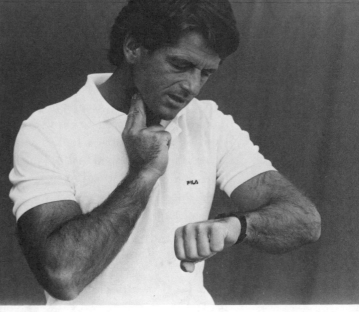

benefits of aerobic exercise, even if your heart is beating at over 65 percent of its maximum and your muscles are working.

Monitoring the pulse to make sure the exercise is aerobic

## The Target Heart Rate

To monitor your heart rate, take your pulse. You won't be able to count accurately when you are at your most active, so first decrease the intensity of your efforts. If you are running, for example, walk fast for a few seconds. Then, before you have a chance to recover and while you are still breathing hard, place your finger over either the carotid artery in the neck or the radial artery in the wrist. (See photo.)

Count your pulse for fifteen seconds, and then multiply that number by four to get the number of heartbeats per minute. Well-trained individuals start recovering from exercise after fifteen seconds, at which point the heart rate drops dramatically. Counting for a longer period of time may therefore be inaccurate.

I do not recommend counting for six seconds and multiplying by ten, or for ten seconds and multiplying by six. You can easily make a mistake in either the number of beats or the time in such a short interval and thus come up with an unreliable estimate. While not foolproof, the fifteen-second period gives you more time to average out an inadvertent mechanical counting error.

Because this measurement is so important, you might consider buying a good heart-rate monitor. The best have sensing mechanisms that attach directly to your chest, as opposed to the more unreliable hand-held devices and fingertip heart-rate monitors. Some of these, such as the Exersentry model, beep at both low and high target heart rates, and can therefore be used as a biofeedback tool. The machine beeps until the aerobic threshold is reached. As soon as it stops, you know you are working within the threshold. Then, if you exercise too hard and push yourself into a heart rate that is too intense or slow down and fall below the threshold, the machine beeps again, warning you to adjust the pace.

## Aerobic vs. Anaerobic Thresholds

Your level of fitness and exercise goals determine which end of your target heart rate range to work at. If you are sedentary or overweight, or have medical problems, exercise at the lower end of the scale. If you are already fit or are interested in competitive events, spend at least some of the time working at its higher end.

To understand these thresholds, imagine a scale of difficulty of exercise. Aerobic exercise is at the easier end of the scale, anaerobic at the strenuous end. In aerobic exercise, the body derives most of its energy from oxygen supplied by the heart and lungs. Aerobic exercise begins when the heart rate reaches 65 percent of its maximum for that individual, or when he crosses the aerobic threshold. Exercise performed at or just above the aerobic threshold is sufficiently intense to provide cardiopulmonary benefits, yet can be performed for long periods of time and is almost always perceived as pleasant.

As the intensity of the exercise reaches more strenuous levels, the ability of the heart and lungs to supply oxygen becomes limited and the muscles must derive more energy from anaerobic metabolism within the muscles. As you ascend the scale of difficulty, then, you go from exercise that is almost entirely aerobic to exercise that is almost entirely anaerobic.

Unlike the aerobic threshold, which is crossed when 65 percent of the maximum heart rate is reached, the anaerobic threshold, which is found on the more intense end of the scale, cannot be measured accurately by monitoring the heart rate, even though the heart will be beating at rates substantially higher than at the aerobic threshold. (Sophisticated labs and sports medicine clinics measure it by monitoring blood lactate or exhaled carbon dioxide.) Also, the anaerobic threshold will vary from individual to individual. Untrained individuals may reach it at only 75 percent of the maximum heart rate, while elite endurance athletes may not reach it until their hearts are beating at over 90 percent of their maximum heart rate.

Regardless of the rate, exercising at or above the anaerobic threshold will be perceived as strenuous. To a certain extent, the anaerobic threshold is also an endurance threshold, since it is psychologically difficult to exercise above it for very long.

But it is really important to exercise above the anaerobic threshold only if or when you are concerned with performance. While the aerobic threshold is always reached at 65 percent of the maximum heart rate, the anaerobic threshold can change, depending on the state of training. The goal of elite endurance athletes is to raise their anaerobic thresholds as high as possible through the methods described later in this book. Their bodies become superefficient then, deriving more and more energy from aerobic metabolism without having to resort to the more energy-costly anaerobic metabolism. As they increase their efficiency, they also become able to perform at increasing intensities without perceiving the workload as strenuous.

## The $\dot{V}O_{2\,max}$

The maximum aerobic power, or as physiologists call it, the $\dot{V}O_{2\,max}$, is a measurement of the maximum amount of oxygen the body can use when exercising. It can be measured while performing many activities, including swimming in a tank, but is almost always measured while you run on a treadmill or pedal on a bicycle ergometer. During this time, you breathe through a mouthpiece that resembles a scuba apparatus. Each time you exhale, the oxygen and carbon dioxide you release are measured.

In the early stages of the measuring process, you exercise at a low level. The physician then makes the workload harder by raising the speed or slope of the treadmill or the friction of the bicycle ergometer in increments over a period of ten to fifteen minutes. Eventually the strain of the workload becomes too great and you can no longer increase your oxygen use. You have then reached your $\dot{V}O_{2\,max}$, and generally can continue working for less than a minute afterward.

Since the $\dot{V}O_{2\,max}$ reveals how efficient your cardiopulmonary system and muscles are, it is an excellent measure of overall fitness. By comparing two runners' $\dot{V}O_{2\ max}$, for example, we can get some idea of their relative abilities. If both have identical oxygen uptakes, they could theoretically enter a race with the same chance of winning.

## Crossing the Thresholds

When considering performance, however, the anaerobic, or what I prefer to call the endurance, threshold is most important. Take the two runners with the same $\dot{V}O_{2\ max}$, for instance. If one has a much higher endurance threshold than the other, the race will probably be one-sided. The runner with a higher endurance threshold could race at a much faster pace without faltering because he would still be well below his endurance threshold. To keep up, the second runner would have to run at a level beyond his endurance threshold. He couldn't sustain the effort for more than about five minutes, and would give out long before the race was over.

A high endurance threshold, then, is vital to the serious competitor. But it will also help anyone who wants to ski, run long distances, undertake a long bike tour, or perform any endurance activity.

Relatively sedentary people can increase their $\dot{V}O_{2\ max}$ by as much as 50 percent in six months to a year. If the $\dot{V}O_{2\ max}$ is already very high, improvements of only 10 to 20 percent can be made. A more effective strategy would be to improve their endurance thresholds. An athlete like marathoner Alberto Salazar, for example, could improve his already tremendous $\dot{V}O_{2\ max}$ by only a very small amount. When he prepares for peak performance events, he concentrates instead on improving his endurance threshold.

Unlike the $\dot{V}O_{2\ max}$, which takes months or years to improve, the endurance threshold can be improved in a matter of weeks. The ideal training program is therefore one that maintains $\dot{V}O_{2\ max}$ and, during periods where peak performance is desired, raises the endurance threshold.

## The Right Training for You

To lose weight, change body composition, or maintain your level of fitness, you should train primarily with moderate- to low-level aerobic workouts of long duration. These workouts not only burn fat and increase lean body tissue but also increase the muscles' ability to use oxygen and, therefore, the $\dot{V}O_{2\ max}$. The cardiovascular system adapts to allow an increased flow of blood through the body. New blood vessels, called capillaries, proliferate in all the muscle tissue, including the heart. The blood itself responds to the training by increasing its volume. There are the same number of oxygen-carrying red blood cells, but they are mixed with more fluid, or plasma. This thinning of the blood allows the oxygen to move through the vascular system faster. In addition, metabolic changes in the muscles enable the body to extract more oxygen from the blood and use energy more efficiently. The heart pumps more blood per heartbeat; the muscles used in respiration become stronger and more efficient; and the lungs are better able to move air in and out of the body.

These changes not only make a difference in your $\dot{V}O_{2\ max}$ but also in your health in general. For example, as a result of a running program I placed him on, Richard, a thirty-year-old accountant, improved his $\dot{V}O_{2\ max}$ by 30 percent over a four-month period. In addition to feeling and looking better, he also lowered his blood pressure and cholesterol count, and felt less stress than at any time in his professional career.

More, on the other hand, is not necessarily better. Richard, for example, was so pleased with his progress that he wanted to get even better and decided to exercise not only longer but harder. I had to convince him to hold back, for the training techniques are extremely demanding. If they are overused, they can lead to excess stress, staleness, and injuries.

Until recently, overtraining was not a problem for the general public. With the recent popularity of the "no pain, no gain" exercise programs, however, victims of the overtraining syndrome are turning up regularly in sports medicine clinics and doctors' offices throughout the United States.

The capacity for exercise varies greatly from one person to the next, so there is no absolute rule about what is too much. Rather than wait until you are injured, learn to pay attention to your body's signals. If you are constantly injured, aching, or exhausted, or if you exercise strenuously and feel stale, you are undoubtedly overtrained.

Other indications are more subtle. A body-fat level below 5 percent in males and 8 percent in females, for example, is overly lean and is associated with decreased resistance to illness and performance. Training programs that leave you this lean are overly intense. Your resting heart rate, or the rate at which your heart beats in the morning on awakening, can be another indication of overtraining. To check it, take your pulse before you get out of bed each morning over a period of weeks to establish your average resting heart rate. The times it is highest will most likely correspond to the times you are exhausted, injured, or stale in your workouts, all of which are symptoms of overtraining.

Another indication of overtraining is the excess production of white blood cells. Exercise stimulates the production of these cells. Normally they are rapidly assimilated, and the white blood cells return to normal levels after about twelve hours. In an overtrained person, however, they may continue to proliferate. In times of severe stress, as in infections or disease, white blood cells proliferate. Their continued elevation during the training period probably signifies a constant state of stress and physiological breakdown. It may be helpful to think of overtraining as an illness, and to treat it with the same concern.

## Finding the Balance

Ultimately, to successfully incorporate exercise into your life, you must grasp the distinction between a sufficient level of fitness and maximum fitness associated with peak performance. From a physiological standpoint, you are sufficiently fit when you have high aerobic power and an appropriate percentage of fat-to-lean body tissue, sleep well, manage stress, and exercise regularly. Your health gets its due, but not at the expense of life's other central issues.

Achieving maximum fitness for peak performance, on the other hand, forces you to alter that balance and focus more narrowly on physical work. Your fitness goal, be it to ski, cycle, or run faster, or to win the all-important tennis tournament or swimming race, *temporarily* assumes paramount importance in your life.

Peak performance in almost every sport, and especially in the highly aerobic sports, can be maintained only for relatively short periods of time. The body and mind rebel when kept at this feverish pitch too long. Professional and elite amateur athletes often manifest this rebellion through recurrent injuries that impede performance and ultmately cause failure. Those newer to exercise manifest it in boredom and burnout.

Unfortunately, children are often unwitting victims of this drive to peak performance. In many cases, their parents live vicariously for each competition, and are impatient for quick progress. They train the child intensely all year long. The child inevitably gets stale and unnecessarily loses matches, games, or races. Even worse, the child usually loses his love of sport for sport's sake.

This danger applies to you as well. If your workouts are too hard and serious to be fun, *change* them. Unless you look forward to the workout, you lose the emotional drive essential to improvement and winning.

The adaptations that take place in training require time. Some changes take place in the heart and lungs, some in the muscles and tendons, and others in the mind. Each has its own timetable that must be respected. The cardiopulmonary systems, for example, respond rapidly to the training stresses, but the musculoskeletal system takes much longer.

The workouts in *Athletics for Life* will help you resist the temptation to overtrain. They will gradually improve your oxygen intake, strengthen your musculoskeletal system, and help you maintain a high level of fitness throughout the year. Then, by following the training schedule for peak performance, they let you develop the extra edge when you want to, without placing undue strain or stress on your body or mind.

ALTHOUGH the content of the workouts in *Athletics for Life* varies from sport to sport, each of the programs uses the same basic training principles. Whether you are interested in maintaining your level of fitness or peaking, you will be taught how to use a number of different techniques to vary the workout and achieve optimal levels of fitness. They are long, slow distances, intervals, and speedplay.

## The Maintenance Workout

If you are interested in maintaining your current fitness level, losing weight, or building your $\dot{V}O_{2\ max}$, follow the particular sport's maintenance program. The intensity will be moderate, and you can vary your workouts by changing terrain or course or by concentrating on different techniques. Because cross-training is one of the best ways to improve at a sport, prevent boredom, and increase enjoyment, each workout schedule also includes optional ways to incorporate other sports into your program.

## The Training Program

To develop peak performance for a competition, follow the training program in each sport. These workouts are generally more demanding and call for an increased commitment. To bring the fastest improvements, they concentrate more on sport specificity, that is, the specific exercises that build strength in the muscles required by the sport, than on cross-training. Even though these workouts tend to be more difficult than the maintenance workouts, they are not unendurable or even painful. Because they are so goal-oriented, in fact, they will help you focus on your training goals and keep you motivated.

Whether you are on the maintenance or peak performance training schedules, each workout has three distinct parts: the warm-up, the aerobic com-

# 3 The Athletics-for-Life Workout

ponent, and the cool-down. However tempting it may be to cheat on any of the three, give each component its due.

## The Warm-Up

As you have learned from Chapter 1, stretching before you exercise has nothing to do with a proper warm-up. Warming up prepares the heart, lungs, muscles, and tendons for the increased metabolic demands of physical activity. At rest, most of the body's blood supply circulates in the abdomen and thorax, with about only 15 percent of the blood coursing through the arms and legs. As the activity begins, the blood shifts and 75–85 percent goes to the working muscles. It takes six to ten minutes to accomplish these changes and reach what physiologists call the steady state, the point where the body is adjusted to the new activity level.

To prepare your heart, lungs, and musculoskeletal system for the workout, warm up by performing the sport at a low level of intensity for at least ten minutes. As you do, imagine that you are climbing a gradually inclined staircase. The first step represents a zero level of activity, the top one the maximal intensity required for the workout. The first step for a runner, for example, is a walk. The steps above it are a shuffle jog, an easy gait, and a fast clip.

In a similar fashion, tennis players shouldn't bound onto the court and immediately bash the ball back and forth. First they should stand at half-court and rally easily for several minutes. Then, as they move back and increase the tempo, they should add the game's side-to-side movements, gradually increasing intensity as the warm-up progresses.

Downhill skiers, regardless of ability, should start their day by taking the easiest chair lift and skiing big, broad turns down the mountains, using these flatter runs as practice for the more difficult slopes. To avoid cooling down on the lift, constantly move and twist your feet, legs, and ankles. Then ease back into the exercise by skiing the first two hundred meters of each run in easy turns.

Despite considerable evidence about its potential damage, the dictum of pre-activity stretching is so ingrained that you may find yourself in situations where coaches, teachers, or exercise partners insist that you stretch before you begin an activity.

The warm-up, not pre-activity stretching, protects the musculoskeletal system from injury. A change of only a few degrees Fahrenheit makes the muscles much more elastic than at normal resting body temperature, when they are stiff and susceptible to injury from stretching. If the coach or your peers insist on stretching before the activity, first walk or softly jump around for five to ten minutes, so at least you partially warm the body and minimize the danger of the pre-activity stretch.

The aerobic portion of the workouts will be achieved through the performance of the sport itself; when advantageous, certain STEP exercises can also be performed aerobically. Each workout incorporates movements, games, and exercises to ensure that the activity is being conducted at or above the aerobic threshold. To add variety and encourage improvement in health and performance, the workouts also use four training techniques: long, slow, distances; interval training; speedplay; and STEP.

## Long, Slow Distances: LSD for the '80s

In a long, slow distance workout, you work at 65–70 percent of the maximum age-predicted heart rate for thirty to sixty minutes or longer. Don't be frightened by the time, even if it is over twice as long as what you are used to, because the intensity of the workout is so moderate that you will be able to handle it easily.

By far the biggest problem with LSDs, in fact, is keeping yourself at this moderate level; the legacy of the "no pain, no gain" myth may have you wondering if the exercise is doing much good. It is! LSDs are physiologically effective for a very simple reason. During the first thirty minutes of an exercise, the body relies primarily on carbohydrate stores in the blood and muscles for energy. After thirty minutes, the body reacts to the lengthy exercise session by switching to fat, of which it has a far larger storehouse, for fuel. The blood, liver, and muscles, which are the major storehouses of carbohydrates, stockpile only about twenty-five hundred calories. Even a moderately lean individual, on the other hand, has more than one hundred thousand calories of stored body fat.

The brain can use only glucose for fuel, so it is not surprising that nature has worked out a system for preserving fuel for this vital organ. Since there is a relatively small quantity of carbohydrate stores in the body, the body reserves these fuels for activities of high intensity and relatively short duration. In long-duration, low-to-moderate-intensity exercise, the body gradually shifts to the burning of stored fats. This transition occurs after about thirty minutes of work, but only if the exercise is performed at low intensity.

It is true that high-intensity exercise burns more calories per unit of time than low-intensity exercise, so many people may find this statement hard to believe. But no one, not even an elite, trained athlete, can maintain high-intensity exercise for very long because this kind of exercise releases adrenalin-like hormones into the system. These stress hormones ultimately prevent the body from maintaining the intensity of the exercise for sustained periods. Thus, while the high-intensity exercise will indeed burn more calories per unit of time than low-intensity exercise, the low-intensity exercise will result in more calories burned overall.

Not only do long, slow distance workouts burn fat; they are also the easiest way to improve the aerobic base, or $\dot{V}O_{2\ max}$. These workouts also allow the musculoskeletal system to gradually respond to the demands of exercise: the muscles thicken and the muscles and tendons strengthen.

LSD workouts are gentle enough to shelter the body from overuse injuries and the mind from burnout, but they are not the whole answer. As champion runner Jim Ryan once said, "LSD is great—for making you slow at long distances."

Even if you don't want to become a competitive athlete, you may get bored with the plateaus you hit by doing only long, slow distances, in much the same way you would if you only ate grain cereals and lettuce every day. Variety is one of life's great joys. To build it into your fitness regimen and to help you become faster and stronger while having more fun, *Athletics for Life* also incorporates intervals and speedplay into its design.

## Interval Training

Although intense, interval training quickly improves both your aerobic power and endurance threshold. To perform the intervals, you alternate between short periods of high intensity activity (85–100 percent of your maximum heart rate) and shorter periods of recovery at lower intensities, repeating the process for twenty minutes to an hour for those training at world-class levels.

To be effective, the rest period should never be more and should sometimes be less than half as long as the work period. Per Astrand, a Swedish scientist who pioneered exercise physiology in the 1950s, actually found that the most effective interval was thirty seconds of work to fifteen seconds of rest. However, sustaining these intervals for many exercise sessions is particularly grueling.

Although you will choose the length of the intervals that feels best for you, I generally recommend intervals of two minutes of work to one minute of rest because these are the most easily tolerated intervals that still provide major gains.

Intervals provoke a cascade of physiological responses throughout the body. In the muscles, for example, they cause a proliferation of a cell particle called the mytochondria, which, among other functions, processes oxygen. As the mytochondria increase, so does the muscles' ability to use oxygen.

The rise in mytochondria also improves your ability to use lactate, which is a by-product of high-energy metabolism. As your tolerance for higher levels of lactate improves, you can work at higher levels without reaching muscle fatigue.

This phenomenon explains why intervals improve performance and endurance levels. During LSD, the aerobic metabolism is high but lactate production remains small. When the intensity of the workout increases, as it does in intervals, you produce more lactate because you increase your reliance on anaerobic metabolism. Without adequate training, the body cannot accommodate this excess lactate. With interval training and the subsequent increase in mytochondria, however, the lactate poses less of an obstacle.

## Speedplay

A Scandinavian variation on intervals, speedplay is a technique with a less rigid work-to-rest ratio. Initially developed to give runners a break from the tedium of their daily workouts, it took the form of a game. One runner ran for a short distance at a strong pace while the rest of the pack trailed him. He then slowed the pace. After a moderate recovery period, he passed the lead to someone else, who ran at a different speed for a different distance. In the United States this form of exercise is given many names. In cycling, it is called pace line; in cross-country running, chasing the rabbit. Regardless of the variation in name, the principle is the same.

Although not as effective as interval training, speedplay, which can be done in groups or alone, also improves aerobic power and the endurance threshold. As in intervals, the work periods are conducted within 85–100 percent of the maximal heart rate, but the rest periods need not be as carefully timed or as short.

In the maintenance programs, the speedplay and interval sessions are optional but recommended because they prevent your exercise program from being repetitive and predictable. By doing one or two a week, you can maintain up to ninety percent of your peak performance. They will also serve as good emotional preparation for the times you want to train more intensely.

We still do not know how many interval training sessions people can stand per week. Although some coaches insist that their athletes do four to five a week when in training, I feel this "more is better" approach produces more staleness and injuries than benefits. I generally recommend no more than two interval workouts and one speedplay workout per week, interspersed between three long, slow distance workouts and the appropriate STEP exercises, even during intense training periods.

## The Cool-Down

The cool-down is as critical to the safety and effectiveness of your workout as the warm-up. First, ease yourself out of the exercise state by gradually decreasing intensity for a few minutes. Again use the mental image of the staircase, but in this case go down, not up, the steps. Afterward, follow the stretching routines that appear in Chapter 9 for each major muscle group. Because the connective tissue in your muscles will be warm and flexible after the workout, the stretches will more effectively elongate them than they would have before exercise, and will do so without producing tears or injuries.

Don't try to save ten minutes by skipping the stretches, because flexibility is as essential to a healthy musculoskeletal system as are aerobics and strength. The flexibility you gain by stretching properly will prevent many sports-related injuries and other common problems, such as low back strain. In addition, the increased range of motion it makes possible will help improve your athletic performance.

For a dramatic illustration of performance gains, consider an Olympic hurdler. Without a tremendous flexibility of hips, legs, and back, he would have to jump higher to clear the hurdle. The energy necessary to do that would detract from the energy available to propel him forward and result in decreased performance. You probably aren't going to be jumping hurdles in the Olympics, but you too will perform better if you are more flexible.

Stretching should be a relaxing end to the workout. It should *never* be painful. If the stretch hurts, there is too much tension. If you feel any pain during the stretch, back off until the pain recedes.

No matter what you have seen on aerobics videotapes, don't bounce when you stretch. Bouncing can tear the connective tissue surrounding the muscles. Instead, ease into the stretch gently, breathing slowly and deeply to help you relax as the muscles and tendons elongate. Next, hold the stretch for at least one minute. Although many people recommend holding a stretch for thirty seconds or less, it is ineffective to do so. The muscles and connective tissue need time to remember the stretch position. This process, which is called plastic remodeling, requires a minimum of sixty seconds to be effective. In fact, the longer you hold the stretch, the more effective it will be.

## Choosing a Sport

All of the workouts in this book result in optimal fitness, so choose the workouts that sound like the most fun, not the ones you think will do the most good. Since you will be working out on a daily basis, also choose the ones that fit into your professional and recreational schedule. Finally, don't work out until you have all the necessary equipment—ill-fitting, worn-out shoes, an improperly adjusted bicycle, a heavy racquet, or antique ski bindings may seem cost-saving, but they are injury-producing and ultimately more expensive.

Don't be afraid to take up any of the various sports because you think you are too old for them. Men and women in their sixties often ask me if they should start jogging. If incorrectly practiced, jogging can produce a host of injuries, especially in an older person beginning exercise after years of sedentary living. Armed with the information in this book, however, you can safely embark on a program of aerobic exercise no matter what your age.

## Setting Realistic Goals

Before you begin your exercise program, set some specific fitness goals for yourself. An amorphous, simple goal like "I want to get fit" does not motivate you as successfully as a more tangible goal like "I want to run a 10K race in three months."

Remember to make the goal realistic. Just as some people are born to grow very tall or very strong and therefore are genetically endowed for sports such as basketball or football, so the kind of musculature you are born with can be a limitation in determining what sports you can master. Carl Lewis, for example, has muscles made up almost entirely of fast-twitch fibers, which make him suited for sports requiring rapid, explosive movements. Joan Benoit, on the other hand, undoubtedly has at least 70-percent slow-twitch fibers, which genetically endow her for sports requiring the ability to contract the muscles over and over without fatiguing.

Training can and should enhance these natural tendencies. I could never become a competitive marathon runner, for example, even if I were twenty, because I have 60-percent fast-twitch fibers in my muscles. This genetic limitation prevents me from setting an age-group record in the marathon, no matter how hard I train. Although I have done reasonably well in several marathons, I have learned not to build my training schedule around setting a record in the race.

Muscle-fiber typing is only one part of the physiological profile we develop when training elite athletes. At the present time, it can be done only in sophisticated sports medicine laboratories. Of course, knowing your genetic potential to this degree is not essential in implementing either the *Athletics for Life* or any other training program. Recognizing that there may be inherent limitations, however, is.

If weight loss is your goal, you should try to lose no more than one to two pounds per week, because moderate weight loss is more likely to be permanent. Similarly, if you have a great deal of excess body fat at the beginning of the program, losing six or more percentage points of body fat in three months is not unrealistic. If you are lean, however, plan on losing only one or two percentage points in the same time.

While it is also realistic to expect to accomplish big increases in the distance you can ride a bicycle, the same distance increase in running is relatively harder to accomplish, due to the greater stress running places on the joints and the tendons. A beginning cyclist, for instance, can train to continuously cycle for one hour in only a couple of weeks, but a beginning runner usually takes much longer before he completes a one-hour run. The best guideline is to set modest, attainable goals. When you achieve them, you inevitably develop a winning or positive attitude and set the stage for the next goal.

The best monitor of your progress will be success—or the lack of it. When Bill Carlson, a diabetic athlete I trained for the Ironman Triathlon, came to me, for instance, he was trying to complete the event in under twelve hours. At the time, however, he couldn't complete six hours of exercise without having a hypoglycemic reaction. I convinced him to separate the goals. His first goal was being able to exercise safely for twelve hours; his second was completing the triathlon. He quickly realized that finishing in twelve hours was unrealistic, and concentrated instead on his first goal. After training with this in mind, he went to Hawaii and completed the event in thirteen hours, finishing in the top 50 percent of all competitors. He succeeded because he modified his goal and crystallized in his mind the one thing he was trying to accomplish. Now, since he already can exercise for twelve hours, he is free to concentrate on his performance goals and become an exceptional triathlete.

Like Bill, you should periodically reassess and reset your goals. This book will help you do that by explaining in depth what to expect from each sport. You will learn what equipment is necessary for the safe performance of the sport, how to avoid the common errors and injuries made in each sport, and what the physiological requirements and advantages of each sport are. Even though you think you know which sports you like the best, read each chapter and then decide which sound like the most fun. Then follow the workouts carefully. As you do, *Athletics for Life* will set you on the path to optimal fitness. All you have to do is decide which path to take.

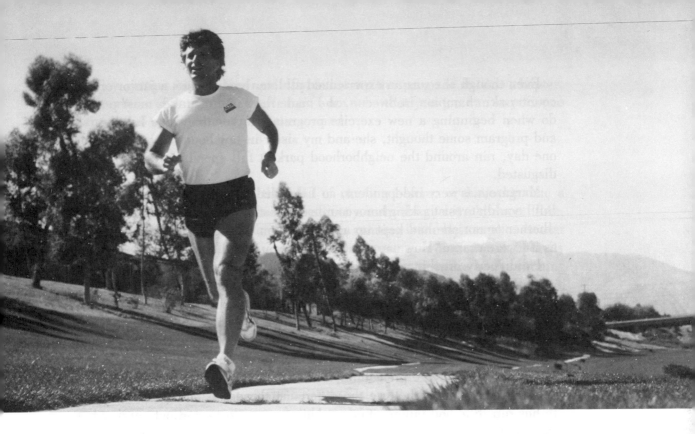

W HEN it comes to runners, there isn't much middle ground. Some are self-styled fanatics who run every day regardless of the weather, their health, or their other commitments. Others run because it is "good" for them, seeing it more as a means to an end than something they look forward to. Unfortunately, there is another group, the running dropouts, who find it grueling, boring, or injury-producing.

I have spent a lot of time talking to dropouts both in my practice and more recently at home. After two-and-one-half years without any regular exercise, my wife Margareta decided to take up running. She felt that it was all that her schedule, which includes raising two children and running her own business, would allow.

Running 4

successful tennis players, for example, have incorporated regular running programs into their exercise schedules. Building a sound aerobic base through running allows the tennis player to more easily add the explosive movements necessary for the game. Additionally, since running is a total body exercise and tennis one that focuses on one side of the body only, running helps establish muscular equilibrium.

Swimmers can benefit from running because swimming favors the upper body at the expense of the lower. Running stresses the muscles, tendons, and bones in a way that an antigravity sport cannot, and adds visual variety to your workouts. In the same fashion cyclists, whose sport develops the lower body, can build up the upper body and derive similar benefits from the addition of running, which involves the swinging of the arms.

Although both are weight-bearing activities, aerobic dance can also be complemented by a running program, especially if the aerobic segment of the class takes less than thirty minutes, which is not long enough to burn fat. By combining the classes with long, slow runs, the aerobic dancer can enjoy improved cardiovascular fitness and weight control.

Skiers, football players, baseball players, and anyone else involved in a seasonal sport also can maintain their aerobic bases and control their weight during the off-season with a well-designed running program.

## How to Run the Right Way

Although we all have run at least a few steps from time to time, good running form is not something that comes naturally to most people. To attain the grace inherent in good running and prevent the body from the numerous injuries resulting from incorrect form, you must master four basic elements: proper stride length, posture, foot-strike pattern, and arm motion. Fortunately, if you take them one step at a time, none of these techniques is difficult to learn.

## Shuffling Along

Susan, a publishing executive in her late twenties, had been active in high school but inactive ever since. She wanted to become active again, and voiced no objections when I suggested we go out for a run. In the beginning, I let her set the pace. She must have thought she was a gazelle—she ran so fast that I had trouble keeping up with her. Also, although she was three inches shorter than I, her stride was longer than my own.

Within three minutes, she was exhausted. "Running is ridiculous," she gasped.

"Then follow me," I said. After walking for a few hundred yards, I asked her to copy me by shuffling her feet. This not only shortened her stride, but reduced the amount she lifted her legs and eliminated her bounding gait. When she got used to this new movement, we shuffled faster. During this time, however, I made sure she could just barely talk to me and still be comfortable, thus keeping the intensity of the effort moderate but still aerobic.

Even though it was her first day, she ran for twenty minutes with no problem. By using the correct stride and not working at an overly difficult pace, she enjoyed herself. She continued with the program, and a year later ran her first marathon, finishing with a time of four hours and thirty minutes. Last year she did another marathon, this time in a very impressive 3:16.

Although many people, including Susan, feel self-conscious about this shuffling motion at first, it is critical to the long-term success of a jogging program for a number of reasons. Susan had a great natural enthusiasm that, as we saw from her first full-out run, made her impatient with anything but a fast pace. She would run like a sprinter, trying to cover too much distance too fast with an overly long stride, because she thought that was what you had to do. This motion tired her out and led to the false and frustrating perception that she could not run for more than several minutes without becoming winded. In shuffle jogging, however, the bottom of the shoe just barely clears the ground as it goes from a position behind the body to one underneath the body. This is different from the usual gait pattern, in which the entire leg is lifted from footfall to footfall.

Another obstacle to her not being able to run had nothing to do with her capabilities, but only with her failure to warm up properly. Without an easy warm-up of at least ten minutes' duration, much more energy is likely to be derived from anaerobic rather than aerobic sources. As you know from our discussion of endurance thresholds, working out at intensities that derive energy from anaerobic sources will cause the body to tire quickly. Susan did not warm up at all, and thus quickly reached exhaustion. Even had she warmed up, however, she would not have been able to run at her original pace for very long, because the intensity of her effort and her overstriding would have caused her to go quickly into anaerobic metabolism and exhaustion.

To understand why reducing the length of her stride worked, it is helpful to visualize how the muscles work in running. In some sports, like cycling, the activity is performed so that the muscles tighten at the same time that they shorten themselves. Think of a cyclist's leg at the top of the pedal stroke, just as it is about to push down. The muscle on the top of the thigh, the quadricep, tightens so that the leg can push down. As the leg continues its descent, the quadricep shortens. This simultaneous tightening and shortening is called concentric muscle contraction.

In running, the muscles are being stretched at the same time that they are being tightened to develop the tension needed to complete the motion. This contraction is referred to as eccentric. An example of this occurs in the quadriceps in downhill running. As the foot is about to make contact with the ground, the quadricep tightens in anticipation of the foot strike. After the foot makes contact, the knee continues to bend. As it does, it stretches the quadricep. Because the stretch occurs at the same time the muscle tightens, the exercise is eccentric. As in Susan's case, shortening the stride helps make running less eccentric and therefore easier on the musculoskeletal system.

There are many other sports that involve eccentric contractions, such as skiing, tennis, and aerobic dancing. Also, some forms of running, including sprinting, which requires the runner to take huge strides in the dash around the track, involve more eccentric contractions than other forms of running. This is important because new research suggests that the number of injuries requiring clinical treatment, as well as the microscopic muscle tears that occur in the course of training, are directly related to the quantity of eccentric exercise. Several years ago, it was proposed that the buildup of lactic acid and other metabolic wastes was the reason for muscle soreness after exercise, but we now know that it is caused by eccentric exercise. This explains, for instance, why it is much easier to recover from an hour of cycling than from an hour of running, even if they are done at the same intensity. Eccentric exercise is much harder on the body than concentric activity.

That is not to say that the body cannot adapt to eccentric exercise. It does, however, need more time to make the changes. Susan, for example, made a mistake by beginning in sprinter-like strides, which made her run

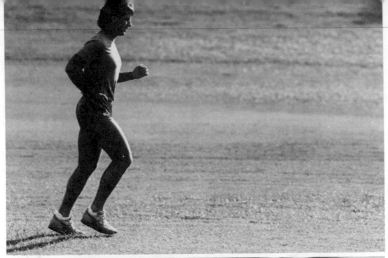

Shortened
stride length in
the shuffle-jog

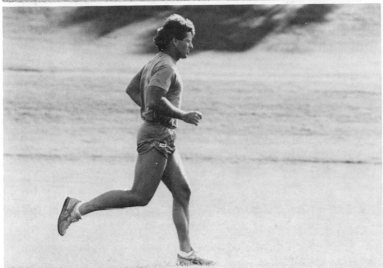

Overstriding.
Notice that the
foot has
already made
contact ahead
of the center
of gravity.

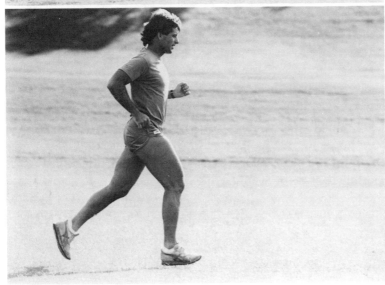

Proper stride
length. Here,
the foot is
about to make
contact under
the center of
gravity.

as eccentric as possible. Not only did she increase the stress on her joints, but she exhausted herself in the process.

The easiest way to find out if you are overstriding and subjecting yourself to unnecessary problems is by picking out a sign post, parked car, or some other object about one-half mile in the distance. If it bobs up and down as you run, your stride is probably too long. To correct the problem, shorten the length of your stride until the object remains level as you gaze at it.

Another way of eliminating overstriding is through visualization. Imagine that your torso is connected to a wheel that moves forward by rolling along the ground in a smooth, efficient motion. As you run, visualize the wheel carrying your torso along with very little up-and-down motion. Your legs have to do the same thing. This should decrease the tendency to overstride or bound, and will channel your energy into forward, not up-and-down, motion as you run.

## Good Running Posture

Another common mistake runners make is leaning forward while they run. Although they think that this stance results in a faster run, it actually drains energy and slows you down. By leaning forward, you place increased gravitational demands on yourself. Energy that would normally be used to propel you forward instead has to be used in part to keep your torso from falling further forward.

The importance of the upright stance was dramatically demonstrated in the 1983 track and field world championships in the Helsinki decathlon. In the decathlon, the last segment of the ten events is a fifteen hundred-meter race. Because most decathletes are sprint rather than long-distance oriented, the fifteen hundred meters was long enough to be a grueling test. The winner, Daley Thomas, started the event with a pronounced forward lean. On the fourth and final lap, he began to tire and unconsciously resorted to an upright position. His body had naturally responded to the demands of the race by finding the most energy-efficient posture.

Bill Bowerman, the coach of the University of Oregon track team who many consider the father of American running, was one of the first people to stress the importance of running upright. He realized that even though people had an ingrained tendency to lean forward, a runner could maximize his performance by getting to a vertical posture as quickly as possible.

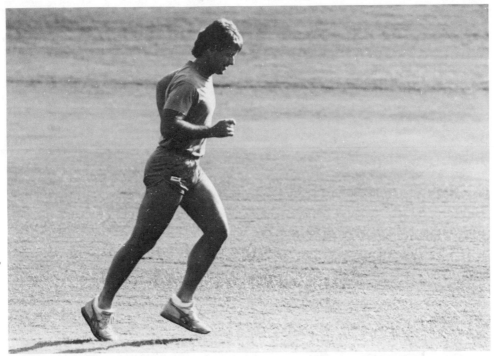

Excessive
forward lean

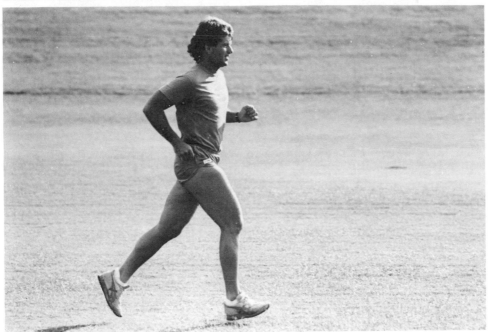

Good running
posture

Bowerman even tried to get his sprinters to begin races in the upright position, but the traditional down-in-the-block stance was so entrenched that even his own athletes rebelled. In recent years, however, his insights have been accepted, and coaches now concentrate on getting their runners to an upright posture as quickly as possible.

Unlike stride, which can be self-diagnosed and self-corrected, evaluating your stance ideally requires a treadmill, a mirror, and a video camera, which you and your doctor or friend can use to observe your running posture. The videotape can be analyzed by a sports medicine physician or exercise physiologist with a knowledge of gait biomechanics. This can help you not only to improve technique, but also to discover the causes of recurrent problems. Running with an exercise physiologist who watches your technique during the run is another way of finding out if you are leaning forward.

Often just knowing that you are leaning forward gives you sufficient motivation and awareness to correct the problem. By focusing your concentration on your posture, you can make running in an upright position second nature. If you are a beginning or an intermediate runner, the change it makes in your overall performance and comfort will be noticeable almost immediately. Advanced runners may take longer to adjust to the change, but they will see improvements in performance within a few weeks or a month.

## Foot-Strike Pattern

Your foot-strike pattern, or the way your foot hits the ground when you run, is another component of graceful and efficient motion. The best foot-strike pattern for distance running is one in which the heel hits the ground just slightly before the rest of your foot. This not only allows you to run more smoothly but also reduces your chance of getting a variety of injuries, such as shin splints, plantar fasciitis, Achilles tendinitis, knee pain, and even back pain.

The alternative, a forefoot-strike pattern, in which the ball of the foot hits the ground first, is advantageous to sprinters because it increases the length of the stride by "running on the toes." You can see this yourself without getting out of your chair. Point your toes downward, and notice how this lengthens the lower leg. Moving your ankle into this position and increasing your stride length is effective if speed is the only consideration. This explains why one hundred- to two-hundred-meter sprinters are never heel-to-toe run-

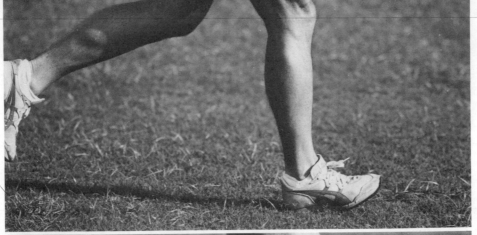

Contact in the
heel-to-toe
foot-strike
pattern

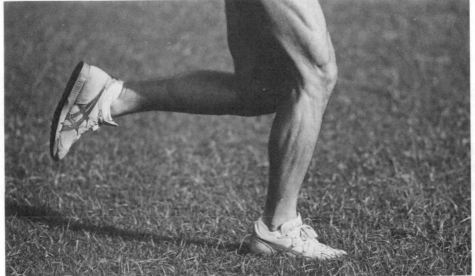

The full
weight-bearing
phase of the
heel-to-toe
foot strike

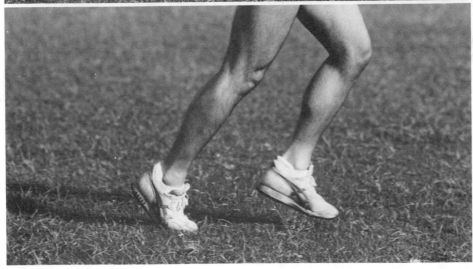

The push-off,
or final phase,
of the pattern

ners, and why ten thousand-meter and marathon runners are almost never forefoot runners. In longer races or distances, where endurance is the primary concern, the forefoot-strike pattern leads to much more rapid lower leg fatigue.

The rare individuals who can maintain a forefoot foot-strike pattern for long distances and even marathons pay the price for running on their toes with an increased incidences of injuries. One such marathon runner, Jill, ran a very respectable two hours and fifty-two second marathon several years ago. But she hasn't improved on her time in two years, primarily because she has had two stress fractures, recurrent Achilles tendinitis, and plantar fasciitis.

Jill illustrates the attachment most of us develop to our routines, even when they are clearly harming us. I told her that I was convinced her gait was a major factor in her injuries. But like many athletes who have achieved a certain degree of success, she was reluctant to change her style of running. Instead, she continues to attribute her rash of injuries and inability to improve to bad luck.

Because the *Athletics for Life* running workouts are mostly distance runs, you should be concerned with your foot-strike pattern. Perhaps the easiest way to find out how your foot hits the ground is to enlist the help of a friend who is familiar with running and who is a good observer. Block out a distance of about ten meters, and have him stand by the side. Then run back and forth a few times while he pays attention to how the foot closest to him lands. By focusing just on that one tiny movement, he can determine how the foot contacts the ground. The procedure demands concentration, but will result in an accurate assessment of your strike pattern.

Your shoe sole may also hold clues to your strike pattern. If the area outside the ball of the foot is worn down more than the heel areas, you can safely assume that you are a forefoot striker.

Pain in the Achilles tendon, the plantar fascia (the band of muscles and tendons between the ball of the foot and the heel on the bottom of the foot), or generalized foot pain, usually in the top of the foot, are also common problems encountered by forefoot strikers. If any of these areas trouble you, have your gait analyzed at a sports medicine clinic to determine if the strike pattern is the cause of your problems. Even if you have no pain but want a truly definitive analysis of your total running gait, the clinic can professionally analyze the biomechanical components of your gait with a high-speed videotape and prove very helpful.

## Arm Motion

Anyone who saw the 1983 New York Marathon got an unforgettable demonstration of exactly how important proper arm motion is for a runner. Although he had never run a marathon before, Geoff Smith surprised everyone by jumping into the lead. At the twenty-two-mile mark he was still in front, two hundred meters ahead of veteran runner Rod Dixon.

At that point, commentator Frank Shorter drew attention to how relaxed the more experienced Dixon's arms were. "He'll start to use them soon," Shorter guessed. Almost as if he had heard Shorter, Dixon started swinging his arms in pendulum fashion from the shoulders, using them to get a greater stride frequency. This textbook-perfect use of his upper body made his running faster, and gave him the slight edge he needed to pass Smith and win the marathon.

Although poor arm motion affects many men, it is even more prominent

Proper arm motion

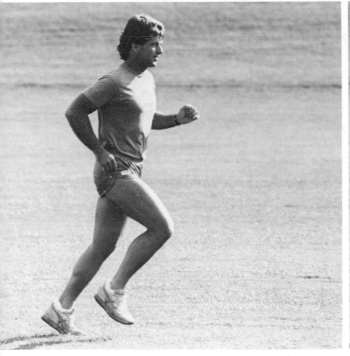
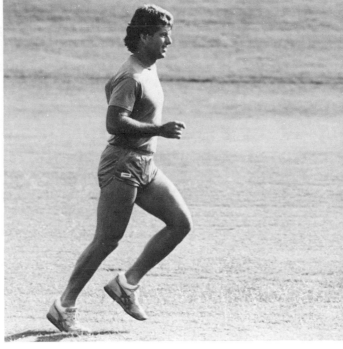

in women, whose pelvises are relatively wider than men's. To understand how this physiological difference affects the way people move, imagine what running looks like from the level of the pelvis. When you take a step, one side of the pelvis stays fixed in position as the opposite hip swings forward in anticipation of its making the next step. As that foot is planted in the ground, that side now becomes fixed and the other swings forward.

This rotating motion in the pelvis causes a compensatory rotational shift in the upper body because, as Newtonian physics proved, every action causes an opposite but equal reaction. When the hips are wider apart, the pelvic shift sets up a more pronounced rotational movement and, as a result, more pronounced upper body motion. The hands and arms, which are attached to the upper body, react by swinging from side to side, rather than forward and backward.

A certain amount of pelvic rotation is inherent in running, but too much can cause problems as well as inefficiency and impaired performance. One of the major problems of pelvic rotation, as I found out all too well, is groin pain.

While doing a study of elite runners at Sweden's Karolinska Institute, my colleague Dr. Evert Knutsson noticed that the muscles of the hips acted differently after two hours of running than they did at the beginning of the run. A slow-motion review of a videotape of the runners revealed a pronounced waddling motion of the hips and increased side-to-side motion of the arms. The hip muscles apparently had fatigued and had forced the runners into more inefficient arm motion. This side-to-side arm motion caused even more pelvic rotation, which in turn caused the hip muscles to contract even more and tire even faster.

This study should have warned me about my own problems, but it didn't. I was in the early stages of training for the first marathon I had run in some time. But after three weeks of training, my groin hurt so much that I couldn't run at all.

I told Pat Cady, the coach of the Santa Monica Track Club, about it. He offered to watch me run and afterward told me that instead of swinging my arms, I was holding them close to my chest. This lack of a swing has the same effect as a sideward arm swing, causing an unnecessary amount of upper body rotation that in turn causes strain of the pelvic muscles and subsequent groin pain.

To find out if you are swinging your arms from side to side or holding them too close to your body, again ask a knowledgeable friend to watch you.

He should look for an impression of how your arms move in relation to the rest of the torso. Make sure he watches you from both sides and from the front and back. By watching all angles, he will be able to get a more thorough assessment of your form.

To correct your arm motion, visualize the right form in your mind. Assume that your arm is fixed to your body with a pin and can only swing forward and backward in one plane. Set the elbow at a ninety-degree or more acute angle and leave it there. Then, keeping the elbow in this position, swing the upper part of your arm forward and backward as loosely as you can.

A good way to learn correct arm motion is by using light hand weights in your workouts, because running with them is difficult unless the arms swing correctly in a forward and backward motion. It is very uncomfortable to run with these weights if your arms move from side to side, so you naturally adopt a more efficient forward and backward swing.

When I was correcting my problem, I temporarily backed off high mileage, and concentrated on improving my arm swing by working with the weights two or three times a week for a month. By the end of the fourth week, I was able again to run long distances with no subsequent groin pain.

Most women should use one- to two-pound weights, while most men can use two- to four-pound ones. Run with them two to three times a week, but at a slower running pace (75–80 percent) than your normal exercise pace. Don't worry about losing speed—eventually you will be able to run faster with better arm motion. In the meantime, your workout will be just as aerobic because the weights intensify the involvement of the arms and shoulders in running. As a further benefit, they will simultaneously develop the muscles of the upper body.

If you use the weights, make sure to use them correctly. Simply strapping them on and running with your hands hanging by your side will not improve your arm motion at all. The whole point of using the hand weights is to get your arms in the proper position, which is a ninety-degree angle or greater, and swinging them as if the weights weren't there. Only when used in this fashion do the weights become a valuable aid in improving your running.

Is all of this, you may ask, much ado about nothing? You're not training for the Olympics so what difference can a little forefoot striking, overstriding, forward lean, or improper arm motion make to your casual running program?

Unfortunately, every day in my sports medicine practice I see problems resulting from careless technique, primarily in casual runners who didn't think they ran enough to give much thought to form. What is even worse is that typically these people have already seen at least one other doctor. Almost always, only their symptoms had been treated, while the cause of the problems remained.

In the case of pain in the Achilles tendon, for example, the patient will be told to stop running for awhile and take anti-inflammatory drugs. The injury will usually heal rather well. But the cause of the problem, which might be a forefoot-strike pattern, among other things, has been untreated and undiagnosed. When the person starts running again, he or she is likely to make the same mistakes and suffer a recurrence of the injury. Paying attention to the basics of good running is the best way to prevent these injuries.

## Integrating the Basics

Working on all facets of your running simultaneously can become very confusing and frustrating. The best way to integrate new techniques is to take some time and focus on each one separately. While you are focusing on the technical skills, forget about trying to increase your distance or speed. This may be hard to do, as a young cross-country runner found out. He was psyched for training and found himself unable to run at anything less than his full intensity. He had some problems with his technique that were also holding him back, and he tried to correct them without slowing down. To his mounting irritation, he was unable to progress in either area.

I forced him to run at 80 percent of his usual running pace, and to concentrate on only one technical problem at a time. Although he complained at first, he was able to correct each of his problems and gradually attain peak form.

With the right form, then, you can both improve performance and reduce your incidence of running-related injuries. Begin by working on your foot-strike pattern, then gradually start to correct any overstriding, faulty arm motion, or body lean.

## The Right Shoe

The wrong running shoe can make running a nightmare. Yet, with so many different types and brands of shoes to choose from, finding the *right* one can be a bewildering experience. You also cannot be sure of finding a trained, sympathetic, or even scrupulous salesperson. By walking into a store confident of your own needs, you stand a far better chance of walking out with the shoe that is right for you.

First you must decide what type of shoe you need. Some are made to protect against fairly common biomechanical problems, such as the inward rotation of the foot known as pronation. Others are made to absorb the shocks and jarring motions running imparts to the skeletal system. Still others are lightweight and built for racing.

Too many people gravitate toward these lightweight shoes, perhaps because they seem glamorous and more likely to improve speed. But if you are just beginning a running program, don't even try them on. Designed for elite marathoners and long-distance runners, who rarely weigh over one hundred and fifty pounds, these shoes will not provide adequate protection for heavier individuals. Unless speed is the critical consideration in the running program, even people with slight builds would do better with a heavier, more cushioned shoe.

If you are just starting to run, or are maintaining your weight or performance or training for a 10K race, ask for a casual running shoe suitable for distances of seven to thirty miles a week. If you are training for a marathon and running more than thirty miles a week, look at the more advanced training shoes.

Regardless of the type of shoe you select, don't consider price when you try them on. It may be tempting to try to save ten dollars by buying a cheaper model or one that is on sale. Even the most expensive shoe, however, is less expensive than several visits to the doctor's office, so buy the best shoe available that meets your requirements.

One way to do this is by reading *Runner's World* magazine's annual survey of running shoes, which has ratings and comments about all of the leading models. You also might call up the coach of the local high school or college track team and find out where his runners buy their shoes. That store can usually offer the most extensive selection, as well as the most knowledgeable sales help. By going there instead of to a discount store that pushes inventory overstocks or high-volume price breaks on limited selections, you are more likely to find a shoe that suits your needs and fits properly.

First, test the bend in the shoe. Hold the forefront of the shoe in one hand and place your other hand on the heel counter. Then, firmly holding

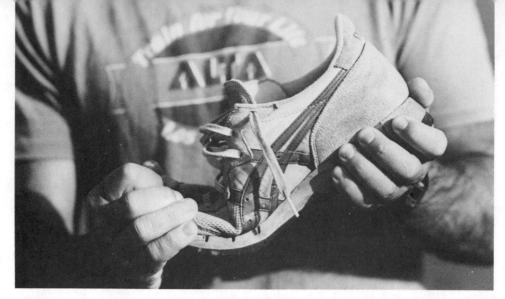

Testing the flex position of the shoe

the shoe's forefront, lift the heel and note where the shoe bends. A good running shoe will bend right at the ball of the foot, or under the metatarsal bones. If it bends in the middle, it may cause your foot to jam against the front of the shoe. This improper bend inhibits the optimal push-off phase of the stride as well.

Next, check the heel of the shoe. It should be constructed to hold your foot in when you take a step, and prevent your heel from moving from side to side. To check this, hold the shoe by the sole with one hand and use the other to grasp the heel cup. Try to move the shoe from side to side. Poorly constructed shoes with flimsy heel cups will readily move from side to side, but a shoe with a good heel will resist any lateral motion.

Like ski boots, running shoes should be comfortable the moment you try them on. To guarantee a good fit, spend at least ten to fifteen minutes walking around the store in them. By the end of that time, you should have a good idea of how they will feel.

Your toes should be snug but not tight in the shoe. If you can't wiggle them, or if the toe box in the front of the shoe is uncomfortable, try on a different size or a different model. People often tend to buy a shoe on the short side, thinking that it will stretch out a bit, but this rarely happens. Instead, toes become blistered or black and blue from the toe hitting against the front of the shoe. So spend the extra time in the store and make sure that the shoe fits properly before you buy it.

Some shoes, especially Nike and New Balance, tend to be made for wider feet; so if you have a narrow foot, these shoes may not be appropriate for you. Make a point of asking about width before you even begin trying the shoes on, and check the fit in this area while you are wearing them. If the salesperson is not helpful, find one who is or go to another store.

If your heel does not slide into the shoe correctly once you try it on, the back of the shoe will feel hard against your foot and, after any length of time, will cause painful blisters. To avoid these blisters, make sure that your heel is still comfortably nestled in the shoe after the fifteen-minute trial period.

Your heel should not be so comfortable, however, that your foot lifts out of the heel when you move. Be cautious if the salesperson tells you that can be corrected by lacing the shoes in an elaborate way. Lacing cannot make up for a deficiency in fit. Don't give in to any reassuring sales pitches to the contrary.

Some shoes will feel squishy and soft when you stand in them; others will be firm. Whether you have been running regularly or are just starting, go with whatever feels best to you.

Finally, turn your attention to the sole. When the running boom hit in the early '70s, there was a lot of hype about Bill Bowerman's waffle sole, which he developed because his cross-country runners were training on wet grass and needed a shoe that wouldn't slip. Later, runners found that when they wore it on hard surfaces, it had a tremendous cushioning effect.

Bowerman's sole was the forerunner of today's shock-absorbent soles. Now, however, the materials, not the shape, of the sole provide the cushioning. Check the *Runner's World* survey for the ratings of the various soles, paying attention to the conditions, such as wet, dry, paved, or unpaved surfaces, that you are going to be running on.

The newest development in soles is the air sole, which feels fabulous when you first try the shoe on. They are not without problems, however. Nike developed the air sole in response to a study suggesting that a rare anemia might be caused by the fracturing of red blood cells in the heel during running. The air sole is particularly shock absorbent and may prevent this fracturing.

The vast majority of runners never experience this problem, so you should consider the air sole for its shock absorption, rather than its protection from anemia. Before you buy a pair of these shoes, however, you should know that they lose their absorptive properties approximately twice as quickly as shoes made with other materials. Even so, many runners who use the shoes feel that the comfort and protection, while short-term, is worth the expense of replacing them more frequently.

Many running stores also sell sorbothane heel lifts to decrease the force of gravity on the body during foot strike. Sorbothane has the longest life and the highest ability to absorb shock of any synthetic material. It is too heavy to make up an entire sole but can be used as a heel lift. While no substitute for correct running form, these heel lifts have helped some of my patients who suffer various foot and ankle problems, such as Achilles tendinitis. Thus, while the heel lifts should not be put in running shoes as a matter of course, they may be useful if you have problems.

## Pronation: The Facts

Pronation is a dynamic motion of the foot and ankle that all people use when they run. To understand it, hold your hand palm upright in front of you. Then rotate the hand and the forearm so that the palm faces the ground. You have just pronated your hand.

Your foot operates in the same way, although through a much smaller range of motion. At foot strike, most people hit on the outside of the foot. As the foot lands, it pronates and the inside of the foot then makes contact with the ground.

Pronation is inherent in running. Many people, however, overpronate, or hit the ground with too pronounced a roll. This overpronation, in fact, is the single most common biomechanical problem of the foot.

It is extremely difficult to tell the precise magnitude of your pronation. A rough guide to whether or not you are overpronating is if your shoe heel becomes deformed and pushed to the inside. Foot, ankle, or knee pains may also indicate overpronation. If you have these pains, consult a sports podiatrist or sports medicine clinic for a diagnosis.

If you overpronate, you will want a shoe with some degree of anti-pronation built into it. Check the *Runner's World* survey and ask the salesperson at the shoe store for the best models available for correcting this problem.

More serious pronation may require medically fabricated orthotics. An orthotic is a device which is made to control the motion of the heel and the midfoot during the weight-bearing phase of the running gait so that overpronation doesn't occur.

Broadly speaking, there are three kinds of orthotics: rigid, semirigid, and flexible models. The best degree of protection against overpronation is provided by the rigid orthotic, the least by the flexible one. For all but the most exceptional cases, I recommend the rigid orthotic. Occasionally, someone with special considerations, such as a dancer, needs a greater range of motion and can't use the rigid orthotic, so we compromise with a semirigid one. But runners should use a rigid model. If the podiatrist tells you to use a flexible model, consider getting a second opinion.

All kinds of running centers, clinics, and mail order houses sell "orthotics," but these products are often just objects that slip into the shoe to take up space and don't control the motion of the heel or midfoot. Because orthotics are not considered medical devices and are thus not carefully regulated, you have no safeguards when you buy them. They look terrific in the store and may even feel comfortable when you try them on, but don't buy them. Not only are they a waste of money; they can change your gait and throw your body dangerously off balance in the process.

I saw one runner, for example, who was running fifty miles a week and, while he slightly overpronated, had no pain or other symptoms. A sports store talked him into buying a pair of orthotics. Almost immediately he developed pains in the sides and backs of his knees. The orthotics changed his foot position so that he was placing more tension on the band of tissue on the outside of his thigh, the illio-tibial band. This increased tension caused more friction between the band of tissue and the thighbone, or femur, which led to the pain and soreness. A few weeks after discarding the so-called orthotics, he once again was able to run without pain.

Orthotics, then, are not automatically required for overpronators. If foot, knee, or ankle pain is bothering you and a podiatrist or sports medicine physician finds that overpronation is the cause, they may indeed be helpful. In the absence of pain or other symptoms, however, they are not necessary and should thus be avoided.

## What to Wear

To run at your best, wear as few clothes as you need to stay warm and comfortable. In warmer climates, choosing the right outfit is easy, since all you need is a cotton T-shirt and shorts. Even if the weather is cold, your core temperature will rise as your workout progresses. It is important to wear clothes that allow the body to dissipate excess heat in an efficient manner and keep the core temperature at an optimal level.

To do that, wear layers of clothing. If the temperature or the wind makes running too cold to be comfortable, wear a windbreaker over the T-shirt. But resist the temptation to bundle up and wear excess layers of rubber suits. A rise in the core temperature of only a few degrees is associated with decreased performance. To keep the core temperature at its natural level, remove the layers as soon as you feel warm.

Wear cotton, rather than synthetic, fabrics, especially on the upper body, because cotton wicks moisture off the skin. Synthetics hold the moisture and begin to feel clammy after even a short distance. For the lower torso, wear either cotton or nylon shorts or, if the weather demands, long pants.

Regardless of the climate, always get out of your sweaty exercise clothing and put on dry clothes as soon as you are done working out. It is sometimes tempting to hang around in wet clothes and talk after a run, but by doing so, you increase your risk of developing an upper respiratory infection. Change first, talk later.

## Controlling Change

A UCLA student recently came to my sports medicine clinic perplexed about some hip and knee pains he suddenly was experiencing. He was extremely careful in his exercise program and had been a runner for several years. He couldn't understand how he had suddenly incurred an injury, because all he had done was run seven miles, which he had done many times before.

After questioning him, I discovered he hadn't run for six months prior to the day he hurt himself and had only been swimming during that time. Although it may seem obvious in retrospect that going from no running to this demanding workout represented a substantial change in his exercise routine, he didn't realize that he had forced his body to cope with a major change that could cause an injury. Not even Olympic athletes can pick up where they left off after some time away from their sport, because the body needs time to adjust to new stresses placed on it if the exercise is to be free of unnecessary pain.

Even minor changes in the workout, if improperly introduced, can produce injuries. Every year, many of our elite runners who train on the street and then switch to a track made of synthetic, rubber-like compounds, hurt themselves badly enough to need medical treatment.

Although outdoor tracks are soft surfaces that are less jarring than a road, they have a built-in kick or spring to them to make the runner move faster. They may seem softer when you walk on them, but as soon as you begin running, the surface springs back at you.

In addition, unlike most roads, tracks have curves built into them. The greater the curve, the greater the tendency to lean into it. This lean places uneven stress on the joints of the legs. Just switching from the outside lane to the inside one, which has a smaller radius and causes a more pronounced body lean, can cause an injury.

An even more common change involves the speed with which a workout is conducted. You may be used to running five seven-minute miles. Then one weekend, you enter a 10K or decide to run with a friend who runs six-minute miles. By trying to keep up with the faster pace, you are asking for trouble.

Failing to anticipate or control change in either the quantity or quality of the workout, then, is a major cause of sports-related injuries. The UCLA student, for example, misjudged the quantity of the workout and undertook a run that was far too strenuous for the state of his training. Moving from the street to the track, or running much faster than normal, on the other hand, are changes in the quality of the workout. Either way, the end result can be a debilitating injury.

Of course, some change and variation will be necessary, but the way change takes place is all important. Those people who are able to work out year after year without crippling pain have learned how to control the degree of change in their workout programs. They instinctively reduce the intensity and quality of their workouts when they feel aches and pains or when they are sick. Equally as important, they know how to ease back into a program after a vacation or an illness. Instead of going for triple intense intervals (see Appendix 3) or going for the burn every time they exercise, they realize that restraint and body awareness are critical to the long-term survival of their exercise programs.

One of the first steps in exercising restraint is to accept the limitations of your own performance. In the early stages of an activity, you usually will improve very rapidly. At higher levels of fitness, the rate of improvement dramatically decreases. If, for example, you can run one mile the first time you start a running program, you very well might double or even triple the distance within a few weeks. But once you are running four miles a day, similar increases are no longer possible. A useful guide is to increase mileage 20 per cent per week up to 35 miles per week, and 10 per cent per week for distance over 35 miles per week.

Similarly, after a long lay-off from running, or soon after recovering from an injury, it is foolhardy to throw caution to the winds and go for a personal record (P.R.) or a marathon exercise session. While you shouldn't hold yourself back from having fun in your workouts or even from working very hard, you have to keep in mind that running for a P.R. reflects a significant qualitative change in the workout. For safety's sake, not to mention your actual performance, you will be far better in the long run if you hold back. Like thoroughbred racehorses, champions must be brought along slowly or they break down. So even though it may be tempting to suddenly try to jump an entire level, the intelligent athlete pushes himself only when he is prepared for the effort.

The UCLA student, who was already fit, for instance, should have taken from three to four weeks to ease back into running seven-minute miles for seventy-five minutes. And a runner changing from the road to a track should spend the first week on the track running the same distance but at no more than 75 percent of the intensity of his street workouts. By the end of the week, he should then be adjusted to the different demands made by the track.

If you plan to work on a track, you will also have to adapt to the curves. Unless you are racing, run on the outside lane, because its greater radius decreases the amount of lean and stress you place on the body. If you are going to run a 10K or a course that has a sharp turn or a switchback, build these curves into your training program, too. Start by making right-angle turns or switchbacks over and over at one-quarter to one-half your usual pace. Then, in the next two to three weeks prior to the race, run the curves at increasingly faster speeds until you can take them in your stride.

When changing from flat running courses to hills or mountains, always be aware of the dimensions of the change involved and proceed with caution. As in all other parts of your workout, become sensitive to any soreness or pain that results from the workout. Don't be like the many runners who try to run through pain, because pain is an indication that something, however minor, has gone wrong. Sometimes it is just a microscopic muscle tear or an excess of eccentric exercise. In any case, the pain is an indication that stress must be reduced so that the body has a chance to restore itself. Running through pain will simply impede the healing process. As soon as you feel any aches, reduce the intensity of your efforts to 75 percent of your normal speed, returning to your original pace only when you can do it without pain.

It is far more difficult to increase speed than it is to increase distance, so if improved speed is your goal, accept the fact that it is going to take a substantial amount of time and effort on your part to get faster. Expecting to accomplish it in a few weeks is not only unrealistic: it is an invitation to failure.

Whether your goal is speed or distance, don't become frustrated by the amount of time it takes to improve. Instead, be patient and enjoy the process of improving as much as the improvements themselves. That way, getting there is a pleasurable end in itself.

## Running in STEP

STEP, or the Specific Training Exercise Program, breaks a sport down into various biomechanical motions. In the case of running, you will need a certain degree of leg strength not found in the general population. Over time, you will develop that strength just by running. To intensify your progress, you can do specific exercises that increase the muscle tension in the specific muscles running depends on.

Because running on hills requires more muscle tension and thus more strength than running on flat land, you can build power by running on gently sloping hills. Running down a gently sloping hill for at least four hundred yards is particularly useful in building leg speed and improving stride length. On either uphill or downhill slopes, do repeats or, if you want, intervals. If you are trying to build strength or speed, do one downhill and two uphill workouts a week. If you live in an area where there are no hills, stadium steps can work just as well for the uphill workouts.

You can also increase your strength by working on the leg press machine. Because the exercise should simulate the running movement as closely as possible, alternate the legs in the press, and then do both legs at the same time.

Yet another way to build up your legs is by wearing a fisherman's vest. Years ago, we used to place fishing weights in the pockets of such a vest to increase the workout's difficulty, but now many running stores have similar vests that can be filled with water to add weight. This is an excellent way to develop strength while running.

If you are interested in building upper body strength, run with weights held in your hands. One- to four-pound hand weights are the maximum most runners will safely tolerate at first. If you weigh about one hundred and twenty pounds, stick to the one- to two-pound weights. Two- to four-pound weights are more appropriate for men weighing at least one hundred and seventy pounds.

Generally speaking, you should be able to tolerate from one to five percent of your body weight carried in your hands and up to twenty percent if worn in a vest next to your upper body, depending on the type of workout and the state of your training. Still, it is important not to start with the maximum, but to increase the weights little by little. Only when you get used to them should you increase the load. Finally, while hand and upper body weights are useful training aids, weights worn around the ankles can alter stride length and produce serious problems. Don't use them.

To accelerate the development of an aerobic base, do a STEP workout once a week.

## The Workouts

Before you choose a specific workout, spend some time deciding what your purpose is. If you have never run before, begin with the program for the first time runner. If you need work on your aerobic base, have only run from time to time, want to lose weight or only slightly improve your running, choose the maintenance program. If in the next three months you want to run a 10K or, if you are already in good shape, a marathon, go directly to the training workouts.

Regardless of which workout you choose, the warm-up will be the same— a brisk walk that over ten minutes gradually builds up to your running speed.

### The first-time runner

If you have never run before and don't think you can, try to run for fifteen minutes using a shuffle jog without stopping. If you give out before the fifteen minutes are up, alternate walking one block and jogging one block for fifteen minutes. Do this for a few days, and then build up the distance so that you are jogging for two blocks and walking for two blocks. After the first week, try to jog three blocks and walk three blocks for the fifteen-minute segment.

As soon as you can, jog twice as far as you walk. By slowly increasing the distance, you should be jogging for fifteen minutes without strain in one month.

### Running vs. walking

Unlike most other fitness programs, *Athletics for Life* concentrates on running, rather than walking or jogging. There is no reason why walking can't be an enjoyable exercise, and certain people, primarily those who are obese, should not jog. But after a time, you will not be able to walk fast enough to make it an aerobic exercise. To make the sufficient cardiovascular demands on your body, you would have to walk with a stride that can actually place more stress on the body than jogging does.

When you reach that stage, it is more natural to shuffle jog, which reduces the stress placed on the skeletal system by as much as 20 percent. Eventually even jogging will lose its effectiveness, and a longer stride, characteristic of running, will become more comfortable and efficient. Because you will have prepared your musculoskeletal system through the gradual exposure to the stress, you will suffer none of the aches, pains, or problems common among less prepared new runners.

Similarly, racewalking is anything but a natural movement, and was developed with rules that prevent the body from doing what it would naturally. To keep one foot on the ground at all times, for instance, the racewalker must lift the hip on one side of the body so that the back leg can swing through while the front leg maintains contact with the ground. This is neither inherently more efficient nor safer than running.

Don't worry, however, if you are not yet ready to run. Just substitute walking or jogging for running in the workouts. Take your time; before long, you will want to build up speed and become a runner, rather than a jogger.

## The Maintenance Program

It is difficult to maintain performance and interest in a sport if you participate only in that one activity. For that reason, I believe that a workout program has a better chance of success if it incorporates more than one activity.

Running, for instance, is almost unparalleled in its cardiovascular benefits and ability to control stress and weight. Yet as a gravity-dependent sport, it places stress on the musculoskeletal system that at times can be excessive. To give the body a rest from that pounding, complement the running with two workouts a week of cycling, swimming, or weight training. Similarly, playing a skill sport such as racquetball or tennis once or twice a week can add an interesting mental challenge to your program.

Even in the running workouts themselves, variation is critical. So that you don't fall into a rut, never repeat a workout's course or intensity twice in a row. If you don't live in an area where you can vary the terrain from flat to hills or from a road to dirt to a track, add variety by reversing the direction in which you run the course. Then, on another day, divide the run into sections and do a modified version of speedplay. Run one section hard, another slow, another at a moderate pace, and so on until the workout is completed.

For a maintenance program using running as its base, a good training schedule follows these guidelines:

*Day One*—Long, slow distance running at 65–70 percent of the maximal heart rate for a minimum of forty-five minutes

*Day Two*—Cycling or swimming for forty-five minutes at 65–70 percent of the maximal heart rate, or resistive-exercise-training routine (see chapter 9)

*Day Three*—Long, slow distance running at 65–70 percent of the maximal heart rate on a different surface, different route, or running day one's course in reverse

*Day Four*—Cycling or swimming for forty-five minutes at 65–70 percent of the target heart rate, or weight-training workout

*Day Five*—Long, slow distance running at 65–70 percent of maximal heart rate, using a different course or surface. To maintain interest and stimulate improvement, do the modified speedplay workout

*Day Six*—A skill workout, using tennis, racquetball, or another aerobically oriented sport

*Day Seven*—Any activity that is satisfying and that involves the expenditure of energy. If you choose another long, slow distance run, make sure that you don't repeat the workout that you did on day five, or will do on day one of the next week.

## Running as Your Only Exercise

Despite my warnings, some of you are not going to participate in other sports, and will insist on running six to seven days a week. If you do, varying your route becomes even more important. So that you don't get stale or bored, try to find as many different places to run as possible, and make sure to vary the surface and terrain of your run. Also, do at least four LSD workouts and a maximum of two difficult workouts a week. A more intense schedule could involve an excess amount of stress to the musculoskeletal system.

## The Training Program

For a training program to be successful, you first have to decide what you are training for. It might be the participation in some event or a P.R. you want to set at a particular distance. In any event, choose a goal that appeals to you, so that you don't settle for a nebulous general desire to get better. This goal will give your program a specific focus, will help structure your improvement, and will give you the incentive you need to stick to the training program.

Once you have picked a goal, follow the training program carefully. Record your progress in a training logbook. Like a goal, this journal is a powerful tool in helping you stay with the program.

Assuming you have a good running base, you should be able to peak in three months. A shorter length of time will not prepare the musculoskeletal system for the increased demands you are placing on it, while anything longer will tend to make you stale.

The three months are divided into three segments. The first, which lasts for two weeks, helps you adjust to the increased intensities and major changes that are imminent. The second, which takes from six to eight weeks, makes extensive use of interval training. The final segment, which takes place in the last two weeks of training, tapers the intensity of the workouts and conserves your energy for the day of the performance.

### Weeks one and two

So that you can ease into the training program's demands, do speedplay (see p. 38) rather than interval workouts during these two weeks. Don't worry about the ratio of work to rest times. Instead, divide the run into arbitrary distances of about two hundred meters to one-half mile. Run them at 85–95 percent of the maximal heart rate, and take as long as necessary to recover, beginning to run hard again only when you are refreshed.

During these two weeks, alternate three speedplay workouts per week with long, slow distance workouts. If you don't feel any aches and pains on the day following speedplay, run for forty-five to sixty minutes at 65–70 percent of your maximal heart rate, curtailing any urge to train harder. If you feel any pain, substitute swimming or cycling at 65–70 percent for forty-five minutes to an hour. Even if you feel fine, you should do at least one antigravity workout a week so that you get the benefits of cross-training and relieve the body of some of the increased stresses the training program is placing on it.

## Weeks three through ten

During this period, remember the basic principle of interval training, which is that the work period must be at least twice as long as the rest period. Because these interval workouts are very difficult, do only two a week. Never perform an interval workout unless you are properly rested. Follow the schedule exactly, giving yourself at least two days between interval training days.

There is no point in forcing yourself into workouts you aren't prepared for, so use the interval chart (Appendix 3) to design an interval schedule that suits your level of fitness. It is organized around three basic divisions. The white section has the easiest intervals; the dotted intervals are of more moderate difficulty; and the striped are the most strenuous. Within each section, the number of repetitions, ratio of work to rest, and intensities are listed in order of increasing difficulty.

To plan your interval work, choose one number from each of the three columns. If, for instance, you are just beginning and want the easiest workout possible, refer to the white section and choose the easiest number of repetitions (eight), the easiest work-to-rest ratio (three minutes to one), and the least intense target heart rate (65 percent).

Remember that you will improve rapidly at first and then more slowly as you move through the training program. Your goal in this training period should be to work up to the toughest, or striped, intervals. Although everyone's progress will be different, plan on working into the most difficult areas of the dotted field by week six and moving into the striped by the end of week six or the beginning of week seven.

Alternate the intervals with two long, slow distance running sessions and two long, slow distance cycling workouts. On the seventh day, take advantage of a technique called repeats, which helps you peak and refine your racing techniques. In repeats, the runner covers a distance, usually from one hundred to four hundred and forty meters, at a race pace and then walks or jogs until fully recovered, and then repeats the process eight to twenty times, depending on the level of training and distance. Some people will run two 880s, four 440s, and ten 220s, while others will run ten 220s. The point is more to sharpen your running technique and improve neuromuscular coordination, rather than improve your aerobic or anaerobic processes, so the specific distance is less important in repeats. If you are a beginning runner, you might start with four one hundred-meter and four two hundred-meter repeats, adding four 440s when you feel you are ready. If you are an elite 10K runner, you might run four 440s, four 220s, and ten 100 meter distances. Increase the repeats in quantities of four here, as well.

This section's training workouts should be scheduled as follows:

*Day One*—Long, slow distance running
*Day Two*—Thirty minutes of easy running, followed by intervals
*Day Three*—Long, slow distance cycling
*Day Four*—Thirty minutes of easy running followed by repeats
*Day Five*—Long, slow distance running
*Day Six*—Thirty minutes of easy running, followed by intervals
*Day Seven*—Long, slow distance cycling

## Weeks eleven and twelve

In this tapering phase, you are no longer concerned with building cardiovascular power. Instead, use a modified type of repeat workout to sharpen the race pace and conserve power. Run at a race pace for three minutes, recover for three minutes; run at a race pace for two minutes, recover for two minutes; run at a race pace for one minute, and recover for a minute, repeating the sequence eight to twenty times. Pretending you are racing during these sessions will help you prepare physiologically and psychologically for the event.

In the eleventh week, do one interval and two repeat workouts, alternating them with long, slow distance sessions, at least one of which is on the bicycle.

On the eleventh week, follow this schedule:

*Day One*— Long, slow distance running
*Day Two*—Repeats
*Day Three*—Long, slow distance running
*Day Four*—Intervals
*Day Five*—Long, slow distance running
*Day Six*—Repeats
*Day Seven*—Long, slow distance cycling

If you are carbo-loading in week twelve, see Appendix 5 and follow this schedule:

*Day One*—Long, slow distance running
*Day Two*—Long, slow distance running
*Day Three*—A two-hour run at low intensity
*Day Four*—Repeats at moderate intensity
*Day Five*—Long, slow distance running
*Day Six*—Long, slow distance run plus short distance (200–300 meter) repeats
*Prerace Day*—rest

If you are training for a 10K or are not carbo-loading, do two repeats, two long, slow distances on the bicycle, and two long, slow running workouts in this last week of training. Even though you might want to cram a last workout in, resist the temptation and do no more than fifteen to twenty minutes of jogging on the day before the race.

If you are not carbo-loading, follow this schedule on the twelfth week:

*Day One*—Long, slow distance running
*Day Two*—Long, slow distance cycling
*Day Three*—Repeats
*Day Four*—Long, slow distance running
*Day Five*—Long, slow distance cycling

**Day Six**—Repeats

**Prerace Day**—fifteen to twenty minutes easy jogging

If you are doing STEP workouts while in training, do only one a week during the third through eighth weeks of training.

## The Cool-Down

After the aerobic component of the workout is over, shuffle jog or walk for five minutes or longer, until the heart rate falls below the 65-percent range. Then change into dry sweats and stay warm during the stretching period.

A relatively small number of stretches will provide you with the improved joint mobility that is so important in this sport. [See Chapter 9.] Remember that no stretch is valuable unless it is held for more than a minute. By doing the stretches carefully, you will give your body the perfect opportunity to readjust to the nonexercise or resting state.

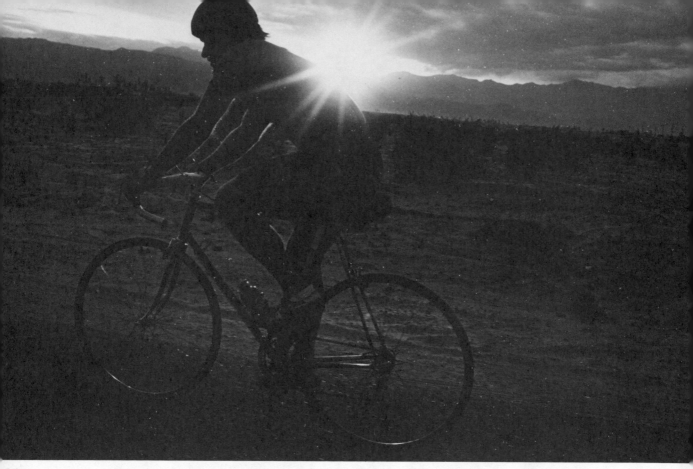

U P until several years ago, people were likely to think about bicycling as a leisurely ride around the neighborhood on a clunky one- or three-speed bicycle. Then came the gas crisis, which reminded people that bicycles were efficient, economical, and dependable modes of transportation; the fitness craze; and the movie *Breaking Away,* which showed bicycling in a high-precision, sexy, and exhilarating light. This new image, when combined with the convenience and overall appeal of cycling as a sport, has given bicycling a new air of excitement and has helped make it one of the fastest-growing sports in America.

# 5 Bicycling

In addition, unlike running, where even an ambitious workout generally covers no more than ten miles, a cycling workout can easily take you thirty miles from home. Because you can go so many more places, cycling is a very enjoyable way to exercise.

John, a health professional and an elite runner in his late twenties, found that out while recuperating from a stress fracture. One of the best fifteen hundred-meter runners in the Santa Monica Track Club, he did not want to lose his aerobic base as the fracture was healing, so I had him take up cycling. He was extremely fit, and thus very surprised when he got on the bike and saw people who did not appear to have his cardiopulmonary conditioning pass him on the road. A competitive person, he responded to the challenge and determined to learn the correct way to cycle. He found that his new sport not only provided outstanding aerobic conditioning, but was also fun. Now, long after the stress fracture has healed, John continues to work out twice a week on the bicycle and would no sooner give it up than he would running.

## Why Is Cycling a Good Sport?

There are a number of reasons why you should begin a cycling program. For one, cycling is an antigravity sport. Running, aerobic dancing, tennis, and skiing all are sports where your weight must be supported by your musculoskeletal system. The jarring and eccentric stresses placed on the musculoskeletal system often lead to soreness and sometimes to injuries. But in cycling, the bicycle supports the weight. As a result, the jarring forces associated with the weight-bearing sports are drastically reduced.

Secondly, cycling is a concentric muscle exercise. As you may remember from the discussion of eccentric and concentric muscle movements in Chapter 4, the muscles shorten at the same time that they develop muscle tension in concentric exercise. New research indicates that most muscle injuries occur during eccentric exercise, during which the muscle lengthens while developing tension. Since cycling is primarily concentric, these injuries are far less likely to occur.

Cycling also requires the use of huge muscle masses and thus is an excellent aerobic sport. It involves all the muscles of both legs, and the muscles of the hips and lower trunk. Even though the arms and shoulders are not used as much as they are in running, for example, it is still an

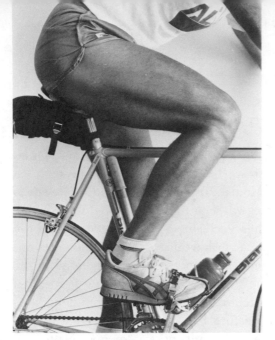

Concentric leg exercise in cycling. Muscle tension is developed only on the downward push, at which point the muscles shorten. These muscles relax when the foot reaches the bottom of the pedal stroke.

extremely effective way to achieve cardiovascular fitness, as can be seen by the $\dot{V}O_{2\ maxes}$ of elite cyclists, which are only slightly below those of elite marathon runners.

As you probably have noticed, however, it is possible to move along on a bicycle and do very little work. Once the bicycle gets moving, its momentum tends to keep it going with relatively little output from you. When you stop moving your feet in running, you stop. In cycling, when you stop pedaling, you coast. For that reason, a bike ride is not necessarily an aerobic workout.

In communities with uninterrupted bicycle paths, making a cycling workout aerobic is less a problem than in communities without them. In busy cities, stop signs and traffic lights impede the aerobic nature of a ride, because your heart rate drops after about fifteen seconds of rest. Most traffic signals require you to stop considerably longer, and can therefore interfere with the cyclist's ability to work at a continuously aerobic pace. If you don't have access to a network of extensive bike trails, you will have to carefully plan your route so that you can ride without interruption for the required periods of time.

### Cycling safely

No discussion of cycling would be complete without mentioning safety. I encourage everyone to discover and enjoy the sport, but I cannot overemphasize the importance of riding carefully. When you are on the road, you are in direct competition with fast-moving, heavy metal vehicles. Some of them don't care about your welfare; a few may even regard you as a target. Other drivers, while concerned, may not notice you at all. Unfortunately, we now think that this has less to do with their concentration than it does with basic biology.

In a recent study, people were seated in observation chairs and shown lines on a screen. While the lines flashed by, a machine recorded the neurological responses their eye muscles made. When a single vertical line was displayed, the observers showed little response. A combination of horizontal and vertical lines registered a much stronger impression. Since bicycle riders closely resemble single vertical lines, it may be that drivers actually do not see them. Many cyclists have had a car move across their path as if they were invisible. Maybe they were. When this information is added to the lack of consideration often displayed by motorists, as well as the very real dangers of drunk or careless drivers, cautionary cycling becomes imperative.

Fortunately, several simple measures can dramatically increase bicycling's safety. First, cultivate the proper combination of defensive and aggressive attitudes. Always ride as if whatever can go wrong will. Be prepared, for instance, for a car to run a stop sign, for a parked car's door to swing out, or for the car itself to move suddenly into the bike lane. By assuming that the car is going to cause trouble, you will be ready for a crisis.

Do not, however, confuse caution with timidity. Hugging the curb in an attempt to be as inconspicuous and as far away from the cars as you can may inadvertently place you at a dangerous disadvantage. When you ride on the very edge of the road, cars will tend to go by without slowing down or changing directions to go around you. In the case of vans, trucks, buses, or recreational vehicles, the gusts of wind created as they pass may force you to veer up against the curb and fall.

Riding in this fashion restricts your options in the event of an emergency. If you are riding close to the curb and have to swerve to avoid a car, your only alternatives are piling into the curb or into the offending vehicle. Rather than hug the curb, then, you are much better off riding aggressively in the middle of the far right-hand lane and maintaining a more visible position. The cars then will be more likely to slow down or go around you rather than whiz dangerously by. In addition, you have more room to maneuver in the event of a mishap. You may have to put up with a few honking horns or shouted epithets, but stand firm. You are not trespassing on the automobile's turf by using the lane, but only taking advantage of your privileges of the road. Knowing that you are safer in the process should make your riding more enjoyable.

Another great strategy for safe cycling is riding with a group or at least another person. By traveling in a pack, you are no longer a single vertical line and therefore are more likely to enter into the driver's field of vision and consciousness.

Apart from a well-tuned bicycle, a fit body, and knowledge about how to ride, by far the most important safety aid is a bicycle helmet. Unfortunately, it is still considered macho by many cycling groups to disdain their use, even though motor safety statistics have established beyond any question that wearing them saves lives and prevents tragedy. Perhaps my own experience will convince you that the number one rule of cycling should always be, "no helmet, no ride."

I had trained on roads in the European Alps for years. I had never had an accident and, being part of the macho group that felt "real" bikers didn't wear helmets, was cavalier about their importance.

Then, two years ago, I was invited to ride in a Sunday morning competition with a Los Angeles cycling club. Since by then I was involved with raising people's consciousness about the importance of preventive medicine, it would have been irresponsible to ride without a helmet. Just before that ride, I had purchased a good, hardshell helmet and wore it for the first time that day.

About ten miles into the ride, I was racing down a curvy, mountain road. It had rained the night before and portions of the road were still wet. One of these damp patches was in the middle of a curve hidden from my vision. I leaned heavily into the curve as I came into it, hit the slick spot, and lost control of my bike. I went over the handlebars, which is by far the most dangerous way to fall.

I tried to protect myself by rolling up in a ball as I flew through the air, but I hit the pavement with the back of my head. As I lay there out of breath, I was afraid that I might have suffered a spinal injury and that I might be paralyzed. Slowly I moved my fingers, making sure I had control of them. Next I tensed my arms, gradually working up to the neck. After carefully feeling my neck and making sure that I was fine, I sat up and removed my helmet. The hard outside shell was intact, but the interior Styrofoam layer was completely crushed, which meant it cushioned a blow severe enough to have caused a major and possibly fatal injury. I am certain that the helmet allowed me to walk away with only minor bruises and abrasions.

Tragically, around the same time, a friend of mine was not as lucky. He was a lifelong cyclist and was active in casual competitions. On an easy morning ride, he approached what seemed to be a clear intersection. Seemingly out of nowhere, a car entered the intersection's right-hand lane, forcing my friend to brake. In the process, he somehow lost his balance and fell over, hitting his head on the pavement. The fall fractured the side of his skull, and caused an artery lying underneath it to hemorrhage. Later that day he died. Had he been wearing a hardshell helmet, most likely he would have suffered only a minor spill.

When you buy a helmet, do not be tempted by the variety of lighter weight, compressible helmets many cycling stores carry. As a study presented at the 1983 American College of Sports Medicine convention demonstrated, these helmets have about as much protection as a head-wrap made of tissue paper.

One would think that the US Cycling Federation would be leading the way in cycling safety, but many races still permit the traditional foam "hair nets" or lightweight helmets, rather than requiring hardshell helmets. Some cyclists have even tried to make the absurd argument that hardshell helmets will adversely affect performance. But nothing will affect performance like a severe head injury. Their claims make even less sense when you consider that the new hardshell helmets are extremely light and offer excellent ventilation as well as adequate protection. So before your next bike ride, go to a good bike shop and buy the best hardshell helmet they have.

Wearing a helmet is the first step in protecting yourself in a fall. Generally speaking, there are two ways to fall—a good way and a bad way. The way I fell, over the handlebars, is bad. It is far safer to go down on your side instead. If you can do this in an actual fall, you will probably end up only with some scrapes on your leg, hip, and arm.

If you are ever in a situation where a fall seems imminent, make every effort, then, to have the bike go over on its side. Hit the back brake and lean over to one side. This should cause the back wheel to skid out, permitting you to fall over on your side, thereby reducing the likelihood of serious injury.

Another important safeguard you can take, especially when riding in a busy city, is to keep at least one foot loose in the toe clips, without the straps pulled up snugly. You never know when you are going to have to come to a stop. When you do, you are going to have to support yourself with one leg. Many a rider has faced embarrassment, not to mention injury, by riding up to a stop sign, forgetting that he was strapped into the pedals, and falling over because he couldn't get one leg free.

## Wet-Weather Cycling

Wet weather makes cycling much more dangerous. The bicycle cannot stop as well in rain or damp conditions, because the moisture on the tire rims prevents the friction pads from developing enough friction. In addition, rainy weather tends to reduce visibility, and the drivers of passing automobiles may have even more difficulty seeing you. The best advice I can give you is not to ride when it rains.

I have to admit, however, that I, like thousands of others, have ridden and even trained in wet weather. If you must cycle in damp conditions, be especially careful about these added hazards. Also, if your ten-speed does not have fenders, wear long cycling tights, rather than shorts, to avoid being splattered with grime from the street, and to feel more comfortable.

Sometimes you run into a sudden shower when you least expect it. If this happens, wait it out under something dry. It is better to lose some time and remain warm and comfortable than to get soaked and have to ride in clothes that are sopping wet. If you live in an area where frequent showers are a problem, you might want to keep a poncho in your bicycle bag, just for insurance.

## Buying a Bike

Up until a few years ago, ten-speed bicycles were all that were available for people who wanted to train on a bicycle. Today, however, most bicycles will have clusters of either twelve or fourteen gears. If you are planning to use a bicycle for exercise, you should think about buying one of these. You don't even have to spend a lot of money to get one, because there are a wide variety of very good training bikes available in the medium ($350–500) price range. A less-expensive bicycle will have a heavier frame, tires, rims, and mechanical parts, which make it less than optimal for training, and the higher-priced bicycles have benefits that are important only to elite racers, who have to be concerned with relatively minor details and adjustments. Also, there is a far bigger difference between the low- and medium-priced bikes than between the medium- and high-priced machines. The medium-priced machine, then, is best suited for most cyclists' needs.

Buying a medium-priced bicycle is much easier than buying a cheaper or more expensive bicycle for several reasons. Unlike low-priced bicycles, which can be lemons, the mid-priced bike bought from a reputable bicycle shop will almost always be of a high quality. And unlike the more expensive bicycles, which have to be put together part by part in what can be a lengthy and intimidating process, these mid-ranged bicycles generally come as a package. If this is your first bike, don't worry about what type of derailleur to buy or what kind of sew-ups to get for your tire rims. Instead, pay more attention to how the bike fits you.

In many ways, fit is a more important consideration than the bicycle itself, because a bicycle that doesn't fit you right will never give you a comfortable ride and will prevent you from training under optimal conditions. Although

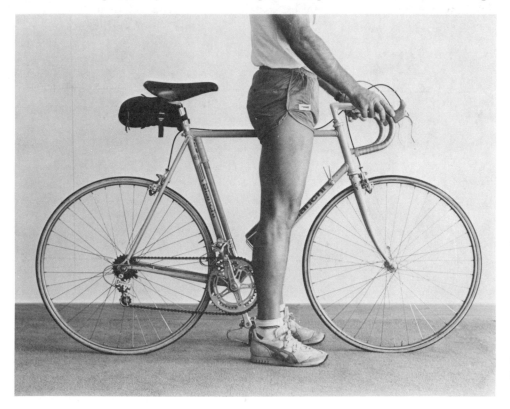

finding the
right frame
size

it may seem unlikely, even a relatively small difference in the bicycle's dimensions can be critical. Last year, for instance, a bicycle salesman tried to sell me a bicycle that was about an inch too big, because it was the last one he had in stock, and told me that an inch one way or another wouldn't matter. But it does. While a good bicycle store will provide you with assistance and should not allow that sort of salesmanship, your best protection is going into the store already informed about what constitutes a good fit.

To make sure you get the right size frame, straddle the bar. Wear regular tennis shoes, and place your feet in the at-attention stance. While in this position, you should just barely be able to place two fingers between the bar and your crotch. If you can fit more than the two between the space, the bike is too small: if you can only fit one or if there is no room at all, the bike is too big.

The seat is another important element in riding comfort. Wide saddles may seem more comfortable, but almost inevitably result in the chafing of your thighs against the saddle. A narrow racing saddle may not look it, but allows normal movement without chafing. Despite their looks, narrow saddles are now padded and comfortable, especially once you get used to them.

Seat height is another vital element to consider when getting the proper

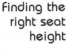
finding the
right seat
height

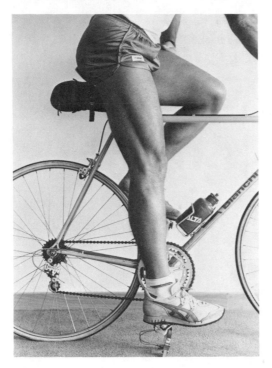

fit. The most precise way of setting the seat is by measuring the distance from the top of the symphysis pubis along the inseam of one leg to the floor. The correct seat height, measured from the top of the pedal in its lowest possible position to the top of the seat, will be 109 percent of this number.

A rougher but still adequate approximation of seat height can be taken by placing the heel, as opposed to the ball of the foot, on the center spindle of the pedal while the spindle is at its lowest position. With the heel on the pedal in this manner, the knee should be nearly straight, with no more than a ten-degree bend (see photo). Avoid the temptation to set the seat too low. Even though it may seem more comfortable at first, it will ultimately result in less-efficient and more-uncomfortable cycling.

Once the seat is set, turn your attention to the handlebars. There is nothing wrong with the touring bars found on many popular bikes, but I prefer the traditional curved handlebars, which were developed to allow for variations in body position, for comfort, and for improved efficiency. When properly adjusted, the headset, or the neckpost that holds the handlebars, is one to two inches lower than the top of the seat.

Do not feel that you then must ride in the classic drop position. In a study conducted at my sports medicine institute on elite competitive cyclists, half

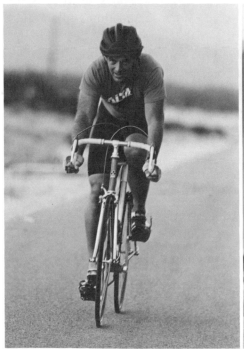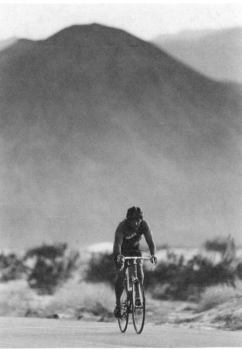

*Left:* Riding in the drop position

*Right:* Cycling in the up position

of them rode more efficiently in the up position and half were better off in the drop position. In every case but one, the riders also accurately predicted which position was better for them. Try both out for yourself and use whichever one feels more comfortable.

There is also no reason why you cannot alternate between the two riding positions. In fact, the best way to avoid fatigue and tension in the arms and shoulders is by shifting posture periodically, sometimes riding in the drop position and sometimes in the up position. Shifting the position of your hands between the brake post and the handlebars will also help relieve the tension in the upper body.

## Special Equipment

It is always tempting to try to get away with buying the minimum amount of special equipment. And while bicycle shoes may seem like an unnecessary luxury, anyone who is training on a bicycle at the very least should wear a hard-soled shoe both for comfort and efficient pedaling. The available bicycle shoes range from those with transverse ridges that help hold the foot in place on the pedal to those with cleats, which virtually lock the foot to the bike.

Beginning riders should use the noncleated touring shoes until they become more experienced cyclists. Unless you are used to them, cleats can make it difficult to get your foot out of the pedal quickly. In the beginning stages of cycling, you will probably have to loosen your feet often. Once you have passed that stage, you will find that cleated shoes make pedaling much more efficient, and you will never be satisfied with anything else. Regardless of which ones you choose, make sure the shoes are comfortable when you try them on. Cleated shoes are built to be rigid, so they will not mold to your foot or become more comfortable with wear. Touring shoes are a little more forgiving, but should still be comfortable when you try them on.

Investing in a pair of cycling gloves is also a good idea. The padding in the palms provides comfort and important protection in the event of a spill. In addition, the gloves also prevent numbness caused by the pressure on the ulnar nerve of the hand, a problem for some cyclists.

Unless you have the hide of an elephant, you will also want to buy cycling pants with padded seats. They are cut long enough to prevent chafing of the thighs, and have a foam pad in the seat area that protects the ischial tuberosities, or the bones in the lower pelvis that we rest on when sitting on the bicycle seat, from becoming sore. There is even a type of cycling short called the Criterion short, which has padded hips that provide extra protection in the case of a fall. This may not be essential, but it is available for those who want maximal protection. Cycling shorts are easy to fit because they are usually made of Lycra or another stretch fabric. To buy them, go to a reputable cycling store and get the ones that feel the most comfortable.

Depending on the weather conditions, wear layers of clothes just as you would in backpacking or cross-country skiing. Unless you are in a very cold climate, you should only need two layers, preferably a light cotton T-shirt and a wind shell. Once you are warmed up, take off the wind shell and ride as unencumbered as possible. (Consider applying a sun block in summer.) The only pants you need are the cycling shorts or, if it is really cold, long cycling tights.

I also strongly recommend that everyone, including people with contact lenses, wear eyeglasses when they ride. In addition to protecting you from the wind, eyeglasses protect you against dust and other airborn particles. It is particularly unpleasant to have an insect fly into your eye while you are riding. And since insects are abundant in the summer, which is the most popular cycling season, the problem is not uncommon. Elaborate cycling goggles are available, but simple sunglasses will do the trick.

To make your workouts more entertaining and more precise, buy one of the new cycle computers that attach to the handlebars of your bicycle and gauge your speed and distance. They are relatively inexpensive, and can help you maintain your interest on days when you need some diversion or mental stimulation to make the workout more interesting. Make sure to get a model that records cadence, or the pedaling frequency per minute, which is an important aspect of effective cycling.

## Shifting Gears

To get the aerobic training benefits from cycling, you should pedal at a minimum of eighty to eighty-five revolutions a minute throughout the workout. This cadence has been found by physiologists to be best in terms of cardiopulmonary efficiency. But you still need to monitor your heart rate, to make sure that the gear you are in, together with the pedaling frequency, is producing an aerobic workout. In other words, while pedaling at 80 to 85 rpm, you need to select a gear that forces your heart to beat at 65 percent or more of your maximum heart rate.

The only way to maintain this cadence when encountering hills or strong winds is by shifting from one gear to another. Many people are afraid at first of the shifting process or don't understand its importance, but it is a very simple procedure that becomes automatic with practice. The gear-shifting mechanisms allow you to find the gear that lets you maintain optimal cadence. If, for example, you are pedaling along and come upon a hill, all you have to do is shift into an easier gear and then continue to pedal at the same cadence. If you don't, you will have to pedal at lower revolutions per minute, pushing down on the pedals harder to get up the hill.

Pedaling harder like this may seem more efficient, but it only makes your leg muscles fatigue much faster than your heart and lungs. You won't be able to stay on the bike and in the target heart range long enough to complete the workout, and thus you will be unable to receive the cardiopulmonary benefits of training.

In addition to sabotaging the aerobic benefits of the workout, pedaling in gears that are too hard also risks knee problems associated with the kneecap or the tendons attached to it. Recently, for example, a Mexican elite cyclist was preparing for the tour of Baja, California, by training primarily on flatland. Then, two weeks before the race, he panicked about his lack of hill training and decided to do a seventy-five-mile ride in mountainous terrain. Not only did he work intensely, but he pushed gears that were too difficult in an effort to strengthen his thigh muscles. Shortly after the ride, he came to see me because of the pain he was suffering around his kneecap. His experience illustrates that even elite cyclists who know the importance of maintaining cadence can forget and make mistakes.

To learn to shift properly, find a deserted shopping-center parking lot or schoolyard where you can practice changing gears without worrying about cars, pedestrians, or other cyclists. Remember to keep a cadence of at least eighty revolutions a minute when you shift. Shifting at lower cadences is more difficult and at very low cadences can actually damage the bicycle's shifting mechanism.

However confusing the gears may first seem, you will soon know instinctively what gear you should be in. In the beginning, visually check yourself by looking at the pedal crank on the bike and locate the two sprockets with teeth attached to it. Shifting on the front sprockets is primarily for very difficult situations. When you get to steeper hills or have to ride in severe headwinds, for instance, shift to the smaller front sprocket—move the *left* gear lever all the way forward—so that you can maintain optimal cadence.

The process of shifting is in itself very simple. All you have to do is maintain cadence and move the *right* gear lever until the chain slips into a gear sprocket. To get into an easier gear, move the lever toward you. To get into a harder gear, move the lever away from you.

Since the chain has to go from a smaller sprocket to a bigger one when you shift from a harder gear to an easier one, this type of shift is a little more difficult to make than one from an easier to a harder gear. For a smooth shift, pull the lever up slightly more than is necessary to make the shift. Then release the tension on the gear lever by pushing it forward just as slightly. This action allows the chain to move into the new gear and lines up the derailleur correctly. If you don't do this, the chain may make a clicking noise when you pedal. If it does, you will know that your chain is not aligned with the gears and the gear lever must be adjusted.

One of the most common mistakes people make when they shift is not anticipating the need for a gear change soon enough. This usually happens on hills, where people often wait until they can hardly pedal before trying to change gears. At these lower pedaling cadences, there is more torque, or force, on the gears and much greater wear and tear on the shifting mechanism and on you because of the inefficient pedaling.

It is both easier and better, then, to shift into an easier gear at the first sign of difficult terrain, even if it means momentarily pedaling at higher cadences and shifting before you are actually on the hill. If the hill is steep, increase your cadence on the approach to ninety revolutions a minute, rather than waiting until you are on the hill and struggling to pedal sixty or even fifty revolutions per minute, and shift before you lose your cadence.

## Overtraining

As we have already discussed, the concentric muscle movements in cycling are very forgiving. As a result, overtraining-related injuries are much less common in cycling than they are in the gravity-dependent sports. Like our cyclist from Baja, however, you can be injured if you don't pay attention to qualitative or quantitative changes in your workout. Don't hit the hills with a vengeance if you have ridden only flats before. Similarly, don't attempt a century (a one hundred-mile ride) if you have been riding only fifteen miles each day. The gradual staircase approach to improvement applies as much to cycling as it does to any other sport; introduce change gradually, so that your body has a chance to adjust to its demands.

## Stationary Bicycles

The stationary bicycle can be of tremendous benefit to an exercise program, and can be used both for training or for therapeutic purposes. People who have been injured or have problems in the back, hips, or lower extremities can do LSDs on it to maintain or improve their cardiopulmonary efficiency while they are healing. People who want to cross-train can achieve tremendous cardiopulmonary gains by doing interval workouts on it. And anyone interested in building leg strength can get an effective STEP workout by increasing the tension or resistance of the bicycle.

I wouldn't have been able to train so effectively for the Bahamas Triathlon, for example, without the stationary bike. I used my racing bicycle primarily for LSD workouts and to get used to being on the bike for prolonged periods of time. I developed cardiopulmonary power and strength, however, almost exclusively from workouts on the stationary bicycle.

Although undeniably effective, a workout on the stationary bicycle will never be as exciting as a ride in the country. Still, there are a number of ways you can make it more interesting. Speedplay, intervals, repeats, and overload workouts, for instance, all build strength and, at the same time, add variation to the workout, so that it becomes less repetitive and more fun. You can also work out while listening to music or watching television.

Another problem with these machines is the calibration of their resistance settings, which show substantial variation from brand to brand and even from machine to machine. In a recent article in a leading sports-medicine journal, *Medicine and Science in Sports*, workload settings of three types of bicycles were tested. Two proved to be more reliable than the third, but there still was enough variation to cause concern.

The sophisticated electronic devices and programs featured on the newer stationary bicycles make them seem very appealing, but these models also have their shortcomings. My sports medicine clinic calibrated some of the more popular electronic bicycles, and also came up with a number of discrepancies. One model, made by Engineering Dynamics, was very accurate. Others were so inaccurate that monkeys sitting at a computer would have been able to come up with better readings.

One of the stationary bicycles, for instance, told a patient of mine that he had burned twelve hundred calories in an hour, even though his body weight and endurance threshold made it unlikely that he could burn even nine hundred calories in that time. He had been using the readouts to determine how many calories he could eat and as a result had been consistently overeating. If you use these machines, don't pay attention to the calorie counts, heart-rate monitors, or other calibrations. By assuming that they are wrong, you won't make the same mistake my patient did.

A less-expensive and very useful alternative to the stationary bicycle is a machine called a Turbo-Trainer (generically known as a wind-load simulator) which converts your racing bicycle to a stationary one. You simply take off the front wheel of your bike and place the rest of it on the Turbo-Trainer, which has a base made up of rollers. You then ride on the bike as if it were a stationary bicycle. Unlike a stationary bicycle, however, you have to balance on the Turbo-Trainer, making it a closer simulation of the conditions of the road than the stationary bike.

The workout on the Turbo-Trainer can be made harder or easier by adjusting the friction of the rollers on the machine or by working in one of the bicycle's higher gears. Some roller bearings wear out faster than others, so make sure you buy a model that is well made and comes with a good guarantee, such as the machine made by Hooker Industries.

## Cycling in STEP

In complicated skill sports like skiing, there are many STEP exercises you can do. Cycling is a relatively simpler sport from a technical perspective, but there are still STEP activities that can develop two important components of cycling: leg speed and strength.

The best way to develop leg speed through STEP is by high-speed spinning at a cadence of one hundred twenty revolutions or more per minute for two to three minutes at a time in a repeat-type workout. Make sure that you rest adequately between work periods. Maintain this workout for thirty to forty-five minutes.

Cyclists also need very strong quadriceps, as can be seen by comparing the musculature of elite athletes to the general population. Elite long-distance runners have quadriceps that are 25 percent stronger than the casually active population, but elite cyclists have quads that are up to 45 percent stronger. If you are serious about cycling, you should consider having your quadriceps' strength tested on a device called an isokinetic dynamometer, which is available at most sports medicine clinics. Elite cyclists should be able to develop a tension of 1.2 times their body weight in the quadriceps, opposed to the .8 times the body weight which is normal for most of us.

The best way to develop this degree of leg strength is through the overloading principle described in the leg strength workouts. By doing two of these workouts a week, you will eventually be able to develop an amount of tension in the quadriceps equal to and probably greater than your body weight.

It is also useful to have reasonably strong arms and shoulders, because you rest on your hands on the bicycle in a modified push-up position. The best way to develop the appropriate upper-body strength is by doing the resistive exercise circuit, described in Chapter 9, at least twice a week.

## Special Training Techniques

One of the best ways to recover from a period of intense exertion when on the road is by a technique known as drafting the cyclist in front of you. As this cyclist pushes air out of his way by moving forward, he creates a low-pressure area behind him. As long as you ride in this pocket, you will have less air resistance slowing you down. To draft successfully, your tire needs to be within one to two feet of the leader's tire.

It is easy to understand why most cyclists quickly learn to love drafting. There are dangers in riding this close, however. The first rule of safe drafting is never to overlap your front wheel with the back wheel of the rider in front of you. At some time in the ride, the front rider will inevitably encounter a pothole, glass, or other obstacle that causes him to swerve. If your wheel overlaps his, both of you are likely to fall.

I saw a dramatic illustration of this situation five years ago in a San Diego triathlon. It was at the beginning of the triathlon craze, when the order of events had not yet been worked out. This particular event made the mistake of starting the race with the bike segment. With five hundred riders of various abilities crowded together at the start, the ensuing calamity was not hard to predict. Only two miles into the race, before the crowd had had a chance to thin out, there was a sharp turn. At that point, almost everyone's wheels were overlapping, and about fifty of the riders went down. Fortunately, I had anticipated this problem and rode on the outside of the pack. Even though it meant pushing more air, I avoided a fall, making the extra effort worth it.

When done safely, drafting can provide a natural rest period during speedplay or interval training. You and your partner should spin—i.e., ride in a very easy gear with a high cadence—for about ten minutes. Because it doesn't make many demands on the muscles or the cardiopulmonary system, spinning is ideal for warming up or cooling down. Once you are warmed up, set the pace by sprinting for several minutes, while the other rider drafts you. Then drop back, letting him take the lead, and you draft for a while. By alternating in this fashion for thirty to sixty minutes, both of you will get an excellent speedplay workout.

Another speedplay variation, called the pace line, requires three or more riders. The first rider sets the pace for several minutes, and then slips back and drafts everyone else. The second rider then sets the pace until he drops back to the end of the line. Everyone rotates this way through the entire workout. Depending on the ability of the riders and your moods, this workout can be grueling or it can be easy, but it is always fun and is an excellent way to cover big distances efficiently. Although you may spend three-quarters of the workout drafting the other cyclists, the group usually becomes competitive and keeps up a fast pace. When combined with the equal sharing of the lead position, this virtually guarantees a highly aerobic and interesting workout.

It should be noted that while drafting is an integral part of cycling competitions it is expressly forbidden in most triathlons because it goes against the philosophical ideal of individual effort that is at the heart of triathlons.

## The Maintenance Program

Since traffic lights, stop signs, and automobiles tend to interrupt cycling workouts, the LSD workouts that make up the bulk of the cycling maintenance program will be longer. Instead of a minimum of forty-five minutes, the cyclist should plan his LSD workouts to be at least sixty minutes long.

An ideal weekly maintenance program combines four to five cycling workouts with two to three workouts in other sports, not just to prevent boredom but to exercise your upper body, which cycling for the most part neglects. Three of the four cycling sessions will be long, slow distance workouts. In these, the heart rate must be monitored on a regular basis to make sure that the workout is aerobically effective. During these workouts, maintain a pedaling cadence of about eighty-five revolutions per minute. Both for the mental challenge and increased training effect, make the fourth cycling workout an hour of speedplay, riding either by yourself or in a pace line with some friends.

For the most part, you can follow your interests when choosing your supplementary activity. Swimming, although another antigravity sport, can be a great adjunct to a cycling program, for example, because it is primarily an upper-body sport. The combination of the two activities is excellent because cycling strengthens your aerobic base, quads, and knees. Swimming, in addition to being a good aerobic exercise in its own right, strengthens the arms, shoulders, and trunk.

Since both are concentric exercises, the swim-bike combination will give you an almost exclusively concentric base. To get some eccentric exercise, consider adding two circuit weight-training sessions, as described in Chapter 9, to your workout schedule. These workouts stress and strengthen the bones and muscle tendons in ways that antigravity activities do not.

Running or aerobic dancing twice a week is another way to get a mix of concentric and eccentric exercise and make your level of fitness more complete. Many of our daily activities require eccentric muscle movements. Incorporating eccentric exercise into your program makes these movements easier and less stressful.

Because racquet sports are more violently eccentric and have a tremendous amount of stop/start motion, they are the least compatible activities with the concentric sports like cycling and swimming. Also, to be good at them, you must usually play them at least three times a week. They are, on the other hand, a lot of fun and for that reason may be enjoyable complements to the cycling workouts.

Despite the possibility of getting a terrific workout on a stationary bicycle, I have not included it in the maintenance program for a very specific reason. The best aspect of cycling is that it takes you outdoors and into nature. To enjoy cycling at its best, concentrate on riding a bicycle outside, using the stationary bicycle only for specific training purposes, rainy days, or the off-season.

Even if you haven't been on a bike all fall or winter, you won't have much trouble beginning the cycling workouts or, as you progress, increasing your mileage. Cycling is such a forgiving sport, in fact, that you can hold off until the weather is nice and then get on the bike without suffering the aches and pains associated with the resumption of a sport like running or skiing.

Actually, the hardest thing about getting into cycling is getting your buttocks used to the bicycle seat. For the first couple of weeks, keep your sessions to about a half hour, or even use a stationary bicycle for a few weeks prior to the cycling season. You will be able to tolerate these thirty-minute sessions and soon be ready for longer periods on the bike.

During these workouts, you can pedal at between eighty to eighty-five revolutions per minute, but in an easier gear than normal. This relatively light workload won't strain your body but will develop both aerobic power and leg strength.

## Cycling as Your Only Exercise

Despite the arguments for a varied physical regimen, some of you are going to insist on making cycling your only sport. If you do, alternate three long, slow-distance workouts with three more rigorous and specialized exercise sessions.

To avoid boredom and repetition during the three LSD's, change the route at least once during the week. If you can't find a different road, at least reverse the direction of the ride. Just by doing it in the opposite direction, you will be riding on a new course and will find that the workout is more interesting and stimulating.

Do one modified speedplay workout, either by yourself or with a group of other cyclists, and one spinning workout a week. During the spinning work-out, pedal at a speed of ninety-five to one hundred revolutions per minute in an easy gear, so that you develop leg speed and, should you want to race, at least some ability at breaking away from the pack of other cyclists. If this cadence seems high to you, just think of velodrome, or track, cyclists, who frequently need a pedal cadence of one hundred fifty revolutions per minute or higher.

The sixth workout employs intervals. The easiest way to do intervals on a bicycle is by finding a circuit or street that you can go up and down repeatedly and without interruptions. I use a section of San Vicente, Los Angeles' most famous runner's street, because I can pedal hard uphill for ten minutes without having to worry about stop signs or lights. I alternate two minutes of hard work with one minute of easy spinning for recovery.

Another alternative is a big block, preferably rectangular, around which you can ride. Work very hard on the long sides and recover on the short ones. Your own particular riding environment and condition will dictate which of the intervals from Appendix 3 to choose.

When combined with either a day off or one of casual physical activity, these six workouts will give you a very strong aerobic base and level of fitness. After following it for six months, you will be ready to train for a race or a P.R. on the bicycle.

## The Training Program

Cycling is not as organized as many other sports, so while there are a lot of bicycle clubs and group rides, there are relatively few time trials and competitions available to the cyclist along the lines of 10Ks or marathons. As cycling becomes more popular, however, that will change. Even today, the US Cycling Federation sponsors time trials in many locations several times a year. Road races are becoming more common, as are challenging long-distance bicycle tours. All of these can be used as goals for a training program, as can, if all else fails, a race against yourself for your own P.R.

Although it still is something you have to search out, road racing may very soon become a commonplace event in fitness-conscious America. A few years ago, for instance, Yoplait's Southern California road races drew thousands of riders, far exceeding everyone's expectations. The Race Across Iowa, which started out with just a few participants, now attracts hundreds of riders, while cycling clubs throughout the country are becoming increasingly popular.

Like the aerobics movement, which turns exercise into a social activity, cyclists are now discovering the fun of cycling in a group. Once they do, their thoughts inevitably turn to at least some kind of competitive road racing. If yours are too, go to the best bicycle shop in your area and find out which clubs or events best suit you. If you live near a major city or a university, you will undoubtedly be able to find a ride or event that you can get psyched up for.

The road races will generally be one of two types. The first, called a Criterion, is conducted around a loop of a relatively short distance, usually no more than one mile, which the cyclists go around many times. These races require strategy, because the cyclists are going around the same loop, handlebar to handlebar and wheel to wheel, at high speeds. Since the circuit is so small, breaking away from the pack is very difficult, and Criterion races are usually decided by an all-out sprint that starts in the last four hundred to two hundred meters of the race. The densely packed nature of this event also makes it more dangerous than other types of races or time trials because the pack never thins out. When someone makes a mistake, it almost inevitably involves other riders as well. When one person falls, he generally takes others down with him.

The second type of race, which is more fun for most people, is laid out around geographic points, such as two cities, or in very large loops. The recent district championships for Southern California, for example, were held on a twenty-three-mile loop east of San Diego.

This type of road race is different because the pack thins out very quickly. Once you fall behind, it is very hard to catch up, so you will always be trying to keep up, if not ahead, of the others. Even though you are on the open road, be aware of the other cyclists and of the dangers of overlapping. For instance, I once entered a road race near the ocean in Los Angeles, that toward its end had a turn with sand on it. As the finishing sprint began, it was obvious that a bottleneck was going to occur around the slippery turn. Fortunately, as I did in the San Diego triathlon, I kept to the outside of the pack at that point and avoided the mass pileup that occurred. I sacrificed a few places by doing so, but at least finished on my bicycle rather than in an ambulance.

Remember when you enter a race that most of them will contain tricky or dangerous portions. Professional cyclists would undoubtedly be able to handle such conditions skillfully, but many people who enter these races are not as skilled, so the danger increases. Never assume that the other riders know what they are doing. You have just as much reason to ride safely and cautiously in a race as you do in your cycling workouts. If you don't want to race or can't find one that is convenient, you can also have fun training on a bike by blocking out your own mile, ten-mile, century, or other route and holding your own personal time trials. Even without a bicycle club or other cyclists to train with, you can hold your own race and get the same sense of accomplishment as you could from an organized competition. You can also train for the bicycle segment of a triathlon, or, if you like to travel, for a long-distance bicycle trip to the mountains, the South of France, or the rural roads close to your home. Regardless of the goal you select, the training program's principles will remain the same.

This training program presupposes that a maintenance program of at least three months duration has already provided you with a good aerobic base. The schedule itself covers a three-month period that is broken into three segments. The first, which acclimates you to the training process, lasts for two weeks. During these two weeks, you will do two speedplay workouts, riding your bicycle at greater than 80 percent of your maximal heart rate for distances of six hundred meters to one-and-one-half miles, resting between these segments only as long as it takes you to recover, or for your heart rate to fall to 60 percent of its maximum. Alternate these workouts with three long, slow distance cycling workouts and two weight-lifting sessions so that you continue to develop your aerobic capacity and your upper body.

The fastest and best way to build leg strength is to finish one of the LSD workouts with a special workout, preferably on a stationary bicycle. After about forty-five minutes of easy spinning on the road, switch to the stationary bike or Turbo-Trainer. Find a tension that elicits sixty-five percent of your maximal heart rate after sixty seconds. Rest for a minute and then set the bicycle tension one notch higher. (On most stationary bicycles, this usually will be either fifty watts or one-half kilopond.) Pedal at a cadence of eighty-five revolutions per minute, and then increase the tension of the machine one more notch. Continue in this fashion until you reach a tension at which you can't complete the full minute of work. The training schedule for weeks one and two, then, will be:

*Day One*—Long, slow distance cycling at 65–70 percent maximal heart rate
*Day Two*—Speedplay
*Day Three*—Weight training
*Day Four*—Long, slow distance cycling
*Day Five*—Speedplay
*Day Six*—Weight training

***Day Seven***—Long, slow distance cycling followed by the strength workout on the stationary bicycle

The second segment, which lasts from the third to tenth week of training, features intense interval training. Choosing the correct intensity, kind, and number of intervals at first is a matter of trial and error. Use the interval chart (Appendix 3) to help you choose the workout that seems best for you. Start in week three with combinations from the white, or easiest, columns, and move as quickly as you can into the dotted, or middle, category. Try to be in some part of the striped workout by the seventh week.

During this time, do two intervals a week, four long, slow distances, and one repeat workout. For strength, I recommend doing one optional strength workout on the stationary bicycle, preferably after repeats, and two upper-body weight-training sessions, preferably after LSDs. Also, if you are training for a century, one very long, slow distance workout of three to four hours per week is a good idea, because it will help you get used to being on the bicycle for a long period of time.

You can do the repeats either by riding the same distance over and over, making sure that you are well rested between work periods, or by varying the distance of the repeat to make it less boring. During the repeat itself, pedal at a sprint pace, which will help improve your leg speed. Unlike running, which organizes its repeats on the basis of distance, it may be more convenient to organize the cycling repeats on the basis of time, such as one, two, or three minutes. An example of a good repeat workout would be four three-minute segments, four two-minute segments, and four one-minute segments. As you progress, increase the workout by increments of four, remembering, as always in repeats, to be well recovered between the work periods.

Repeats should be used primarily to develop leg speed and technique, as opposed to aerobic and anaerobic power, which are best developed in interval workouts. A strength workout on the stationary bicycle after repeats is particularly effective, because strength gains are maximized when the muscles are overloaded while in a condition of mild fatique.

The workouts for the third to tenth weeks should be scheduled as follows:

***Day One***—Long, slow distance cycling, with optional upper-body weight training

**Day Two**—Intervals

**Day Three**—Long, slow distance cycling

**Day Four**—Repeats, with optional strength workout on the stationary bicycle

**Day Five**—Long, slow distance cycling, with optional upper-body weight training

**Day Six**—Intervals

**Day Seven**—Long, slow distance or very long, slow distance cycling

In the eleventh and twelfth weeks, taper the intensity of the workouts. In the eleventh week, do one interval at the first of the week, a repeat in the middle, and a speedplay at the end, alternating them with long, slow distances. If you are training for a century, replace one of the long, slow distances with a very long, slow distance workout.

Week eleven's training schedule should be as follows:

**Day One**—Intervals

**Day Two**—Long, slow distance cycling

**Day Three**—Repeats

**Day Four**—Long, slow distance cycling

**Day Five**—Speedplay

**Day Six**—Long, slow distance or, if training for a century, very long, slow distance cycling

**Day Seven**—Long, slow distance cycling

In the final week, do one speedplay at the first of the week and two repeat workouts, alternating them with three long, slow distances, one of which should be two hours in length. If you are training for a century, replace two of the long, slow distances with two very long, slow distances. If you are carbo-loading (see Appendix 5), modify the schedule by doing long, slow distances the first three days of the week, which is the protein/fat phase. On the fourth and sixth day, do repeats, and on the fifth, a long, slow distance.

As hard as it will be, everyone should relax and take the day before the race or event off entirely and relax. It works.

The twelfth week's schedule should be as follows:

**Day One**—Speedplay

***Day Two***—Long, slow distance or, if training for a century, very long, slow distance cycling

***Day Three***—Repeats

***Day Four***—Long, slow distance cycling, two hours in length

***Day Five***—Repeats

***Day Six***—Long, slow distance or, if training for a century, very long, slow distance cycling

***Day Seven***—Relax

If you are carbo-loading on week twelve, the schedule will be:

***Day One through Day Three***—Long, slow distance cycling

***Day Four***—Repeats

***Day Five***—Long, slow distance cycling

***Day Six***—Easy repeats

***Day Seven***—Relax

## The Cool-Down

After the aerobic portion of the workout is over, cool down by cycling at a low intensity for five to ten minutes and then perform at least the back and lower body stretches described on pages 189–91.

## A Special Note on Centuries

Training for centuries is a lot like training for marathons, because the event takes hours and requires ultra-endurance conditioning. The winning time in the average century is about three-and-a-half hours as opposed to the two hours plus required for a marathon, but the amount of exertion is approximately the same because of cycling's antigravity nature.

Like the marathon, the best way to train for the century is not by trying to amass mileage but by doing a lot of specific training, including strength workouts, intervals, repeats, and one very long, slow-distance ride a week, just so you get used to the feeling of being on the bicycle for several hours. Concentrate on time, not distance, in these workouts, because you will be able to cover more distance in the same amount of time with every passing week. When I was training for a century, for example, I only rode thirty miles in my first VLSD workout, but did almost forty in the same amount of time the week later. It's quality that counts, not quantity.

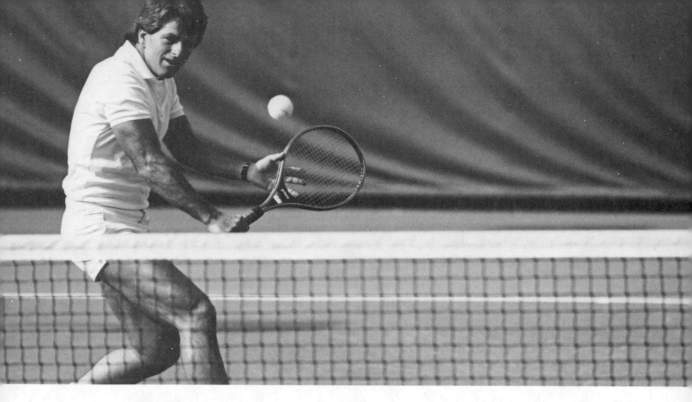

T is unfortunate that the racquet sport that offers the best aerobic workout is the least popular in America. Badminton, far more than tennis, squash, or racquetball, is the most vigorous and aerobically demanding of the racquet sports when played traditionally on an indoor court.

As anyone who has seen it played competitively knows, badminton has nothing to do with the languid game played over a flimsy net haphazardly hung between two trees in the backyard. Instead, it has intense rallies which usually last for several minutes. What makes the game really demanding is that all four corners of the court are used in virtually every one of these rallies. This is in direct contrast to tennis, where most play by far is from the baseline, with the players moving from side to side. The situations are similar in racquetball and squash, where the players stand and move primarily near the back of the court.

# 6 Racquet Sports

Given America's love for aerobic fitness, the game's more modest space requirements, and the ease with which badminton can be learned, it is surprising that it has not become more popular. Rather than wait for this to happen, however, this chapter will show you how to make America's favorite racquet sports more aerobic. In the process, you will learn patterns of play that will help you not only win matches but also avoid injury.

## Tennis

Tennis, long the sport of kings, has a special glamour. It was played in the aristocratic backyards of Victorian England and centuries earlier by French royalty, who gave the game its name, *tennis*. It came to America at the turn of the century, and by the twenties was enjoying a golden era, with players like Bill Tilden and the French Musketeers—Cochet, Lacoste, Borota, and Brugnon—dominating the game and capturing the public's fancy.

It was not until the sixties and seventies, however, that tennis became a truly mass sport. This was the era when the Canadian Air Force 5BX program and Dr. Ken Cooper's adaptation of it, "aerobics," were popularized. The cults of leisure time and self-improvement also created an interest in fitness and sports. Tennis, with its traditional appeal, was perfectly situated to reap the benefits of this interest. When tennis went "open" at the U.S. Open in 1968, allowing amateurs and professionals to compete together, a tremendous surge of new recruits were drawn to the game.

Tennis has the added attraction of being a polite way to declare war. You can beat the ball as hard as you want, the only sanction being the loss of a point. Occasionally, a player even bashes the ball at his opponent, an unsportsmanlike act that nevertheless emphasizes the warrior nature of this supposedly civilized gentleman and lady's game.

Tennis's popularity has tapered off a bit lately, both because of the competition provided by other sports and the necessity of scheduling games so carefully. In more leisurely times, people went to the tennis club late in the afternoon, casually chatted over a cup of tea, and eventually ambled into a game. Now, however, our crowded lives usually dictate our showing up with a partner at a prearranged time to claim a reserved court.

These time constrictions even caused me to curtail my involvement with the sport two years ago, when I began writing this book in my "spare time."

After canceling several tennis dates at the last minute because of my over-booked schedule, I realized I would have to switch to other exercises or I would soon have few friends.

### Making it aerobic and safe

Many people make the time to play this great sport, however, only to get on the court and bash the ball around without having an aerobic workout. No doubt a big reason for this is the notion that hitting blistering placements is the way to winning tennis. Actually, tennis matches are won not by hitting winners but by avoiding hitting losers.

By far the most important opponent anyone has during a game is the net, which accounts for most of the errors, or losers, made when the ball is returned from a difficult position. Instead of lobbing, or hitting cross court, which would keep the ball in play, most players typically go for broke with an attempted (and usually unsuccessful) winner.

This tendency keeps most club players from having an aerobic game of tennis, not to mention from winning the game. By contrast, recall the great matches of Bjorn Borg, who knew he could win more consistently by keeping the ball in play until his opponent missed. This attitude will give you, too, a more successful strategy. It will also keep the ball in play longer, thus making your tennis more aerobic. To develop this attitude, the workouts in this chapter feature drills that improve your ability not only to hit percentage shots, but also to hit more of them.

One of the best ways to improve is to begin every match with one-half hour of drills that not only warm you up but program a winning pattern of play you will carry into the game itself. Professional tennis players use this technique before a match, spending an hour or more practicing patterned drills and finishing off with anything from a few games to a couple of sets. Instead of getting on the court and banging a ball for a few minutes, get into the habit of performing drills before you play.

For the drills to work, find a player of your own or of slightly superior ability. If you are either much worse or much better than your opponent, you won't be able to keep the ball in play long enough to improve either your fitness or your play.

Needless to say, while a game of doubles is great fun, it is not the preferred way to play if you want to get good aerobic benefits. Use doubles as recreation only.

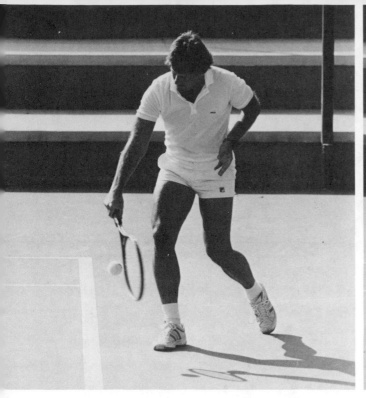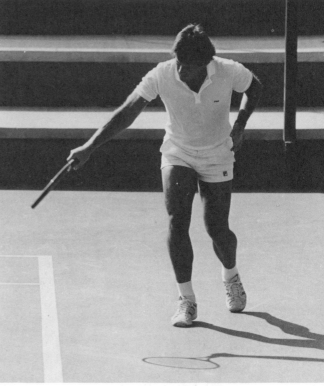

Generally speaking, whether you play doubles or singles, tennis is a very safe sport. There are, however, several problems and injuries that can arise, the most common being tennis elbow. In classic tennis elbow, a pain is felt on the outside of the arm at the elbow. It is usually caused by problems related to the backhand. Biomechanical studies have shown that professional tennis players have their elbows and wrists slightly bent when they hit a backhand ball. It is only after contact that they straighten their arms out completely for the follow-through.

Unlike the professionals, many recreational tennis players tend to rigidly lock their arms before making contact on the backhand. When contact is made, their elbow bends with the impact and then hyperextends as the follow-through continues. This repetitive hyperextension, which is eccentric in nature, can cause a strain or slight tearing of the tendons on the outside of the elbow. Not everyone who hits the ball this way gets tennis elbow, just like not everyone who sits in the sun gets skin cancer. As with sun worshiping, however, hitting the ball this way increases the risks of tennis elbow.

A second kind of tennis elbow manifests itself with pain on the inside of the elbow. This type involves the flexor tendons, which are used mostly on the forehand and especially on the serve and overhead motions. Although it is less common, it is equally painful.

*Left:* The biomechanics of tennis. The elbow and wrist are slightly flexed and the hand is ahead of the ball on impact.

*Right:* Extension or straightening of the wrist and elbow on follow-through

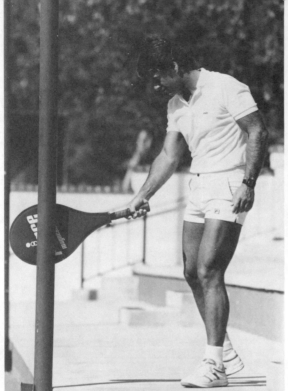

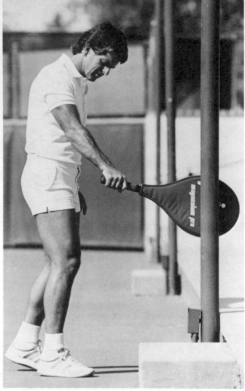

*Above left:*
The isometric
forehand
exercise

*Above right:*
The isometric
backhand
exercise

*Left:* The
isometric serve
and overhand
exercise

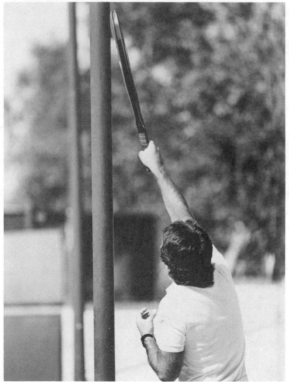

To treat both types of tennis elbow, I use a machine which produces a pulsing electromagnetic field. Not yet readily available in this country, I have found it more beneficial than either anti-inflammatory medicines or steroid injections. But none of the treatments is the whole answer.

Neither is complete rest, which, though commonly advised, can be deleterious. Rest tends to weaken the musculoskeletal system and make it more susceptible to new injuries once the game is resumed. It is foolish to play through pain, but even at tennis elbow's very painful stages, there are certain isometric exercises you can do to maintain or even improve your strength. The exercises are safe, because they do not involve any motion.

Put the cover on your racquet and hold it as if you were going to hit a ball. Stand near a pole or a doorjamb and press the racquet against it, pretending that you are hitting a backhand. Firmly grip the racquet and attempt to force your hand forward as if you were making the stroke. Hold this position firmly for fifteen seconds. Repeat this exercise five to ten times a day.

Next, turn the other way, holding the racquet as if you were hitting a forehand. Repeat the exercise. Then hold it overhead against a doorjamb, getting down on your knees if necessary, and isometrically practice the serve or overhead motion. This sequence of exercises trains the muscles for the instant of ball contact, the most stressful movement in tennis.

Finally, take tennis lessons with a good professional. Your stroke doesn't have to be perfect, but learning sound mechanics can certainly help avoid tennis elbow as well as other common tennis maladies.

Wrist sprains, problems with the deep shoulder muscles called the rotator cuff, and other arm and shoulder problems can be helped or prevented through a STEP exercise that builds the strength of these muscles. Put the racquet cover on the racquet. To add weight, place a book inside it. Using the weighted racquet, practice each stroke (forehand, backhand, serve, and volley) about twenty-five times each. Follow each exercise sequence with a fifteen-second isometric exercise. After the twenty-five forehand swings, for example, do an isometric forehand exercise for fifteen seconds.

If you can do any exercise more that thirty times without fatiguing, you need to add a heavier book or place lead tape around the racquet's frame. If you can do the exercise less than twenty times, you need to reduce the weight. Do these exercises daily, and you'll be astonished at how much stronger you will be in only a month.

Back-related problems are not only common in tennis, but have been the bane of many illustrious players. The career of Australian Lew Hoad, acknowledged as one of the greatest talents in the game's history, was sabotaged by back problems. More recently Tracy Austin, the young Californian who had risen to the top of the game quickly, had her progress stopped by back problems. Even the great Rod Laver might have dominated the game for a few more years had it not been for his bad back.

What is it about tennis that causes these back problems? In a word, disequilibrium. Tennis, after all, is played primarily with one side of the body. While many people talked about Rod Laver's giant left arm compared to his right, no one ever mentioned how much larger one side of his lower back was compared to the other, even though the same sort of disequilibrium was probably present.

You don't have to be Rod Laver to have this happen to you. I regularly see amateur tennis players, some of high school age, whose spinal muscles are grossly overdeveloped on one side. A right-handed player will have an overdeveloped left lower back, and a left-handed player will have an overdeveloped right lower back. In and of itself, this will not guarantee an injury, but it does make the person more susceptible to one, because the relatively weaker side can be strained.

Even minor back strains are troublesome because it is very difficult to give the back any rest. You can work around injured elbows, knees, and shoulders, but the back is used in virtually all daily activities. Furthermore, while complete rest is unquestionably important for a few days in the most symptomatic periods, continuous rest is not without drawbacks. When muscles and tendons are not used, they atrophy or weaken, which makes them more susceptible to new injuries.

The best solution to low back pain is prevention, which can be accomplished by performing trunk exercises. Up to 80 percent of adults will suffer debilitating back pain at some time in their lives, so these exercises should be done by everyone, not just tennis players.

The trunk, or that part of the body between the pelvis and the shoulders, can move the spine in three planes: forward and backward, side to side, and in rotation, as in twisting. To strengthen the trunk muscles, resistance exercises should be done in all three planes of motion. It is interesting to note, however, that none of the companies developing exercise equipment has come up with an apparatus that successfully exercises the trunk in all its planes of motion. Until they do, a slant board and a Roman chair can go a long way toward strengthening the back and alleviating back problems.

Using the slant board, do oblique sit-ups. With your hands on your chest and your knees slightly bent, do one straight-back sit-up, then one to each side, using a twisting motion of the torso as you come back up. Raise the

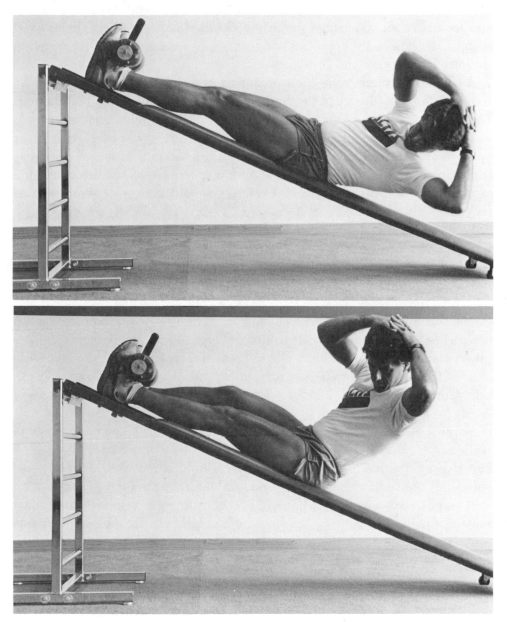

Oblique sit-ups

slant board to a level in which you can do no more than twenty-five sit-ups. As you get stronger, make the exercise more difficult by raising the slant board, by moving your hands from your chest to behind your head, or by holding books or weights in your hands either on your chest or behind your head. Do these sit-ups once a day. Unlike the crunch-type sit-ups advocated at most health clubs and aerobics classes, these sit-ups take your abdominal and accessory spinal muscles through their full range of motion. The oblique sit-ups are especially important for tennis players because of the twisting motions of the serve and overhead.

After doing exercises for the abdominals and the front side of the trunk, you must now do the same for the back so that equilibrium is maintained. This is an important, if often overlooked, training principle, because muscle imbalance can increase your susceptibility to injuries. If you exercise your thigh or quadriceps muscles, for instance, you should also exercise your hamstrings, which are the equilibrating group of muscles on the back side of the upper leg. Similarly, back exercises should always be done in conjunction with abdominal exercises.

To do these exercises, use the Roman chair, an apparatus that is readily available in many health clubs. Perform them in a slow, controlled fashion, especially on the downward, or eccentric, motion, to avoid muscle strain. As you get stronger, you can perform the exercises more vigorously.

Lying face down on it, secure the back of your ankles and rest your upper thighs and hips against the padded supports. Allow your trunk to hang down toward the ground so that your trunk and legs, which are straight, form a ninety-degree angle with each other. From this position, do the same exercises that you did for sit-ups, only in reverse. First do a straight "back-up." Then do one to each side, twisting as you attempt to raise your back as far up as you can.

As in the sit-ups, be sure to take your back through a complete range of motion. If you do not have access to a Roman chair, a reasonable but less-effective alternative is a rowing machine, which, when used correctly, involves all the trunk muscles and therefore develops strength in the trunk.

If you already have low back pain, first consult your physician to find out the exact nature of your problem. Muscular strain is by far the most common problem, but whatever the cause, these exercises can be helpful rehabilitation. However, as with tennis elbow or other musculoskeletal injuries, if you are acutely symptomatic, your first exercises should be isometric, rather

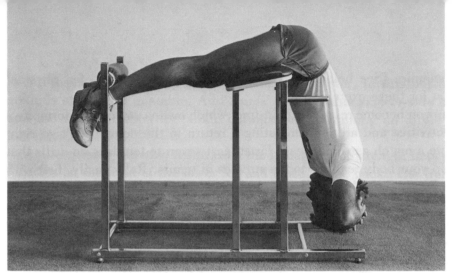

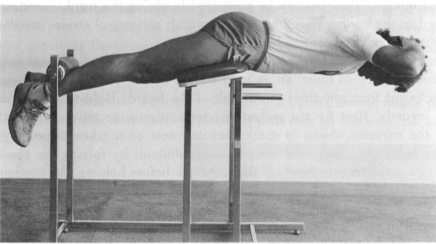

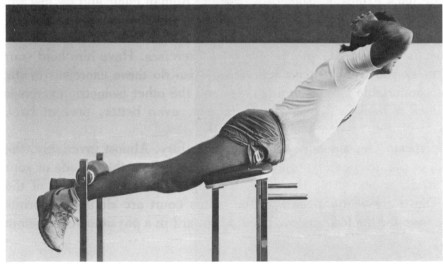

Difficult back
extension
exercises on
the Roman
chair

sudden push-off from the front foot during the service motion usually produces a strong eccentric strain on the tendon. Like back pain, it can be especially troublesome because the ankle is used so much in our ordinary lives. Thus, once present, Achilles tendinitis is often difficult to get rid of.

The best way to avoid the problem is by controlling change in your game. If you play only a few times a week, don't expect to play competitive matches for an entire day without becoming susceptible to an injury. You need to prepare for such a dramatic jump in the quantity and intensity of play.

I treat Achilles tendinitis with electromagnetic field therapy and find it more effective than the traditional treatments of rest (sometimes involving a cast) and anti-inflammatory medications. Isometric exercises involving plantar flexion and dorsi flexion of the ankle (that is, pointing it up and down) also should be done while the injury is healing. For the plantar flexion exercises, sit on the floor with one leg bent and the other leg outstretched over it. The sole of your shoe on the outstretched leg should be flat against a wall. Attempt to point your toes, doing an isometric exercise against the immovable resistance of the wall. For dorsi flexion, do the penguin walk. Like the other isometrics, do as many sets as it takes to produce comfortable fatigue.

No matter how badly you want to get out on the court, don't try to play through Achilles tendinitis, because you will only make the problem worse.

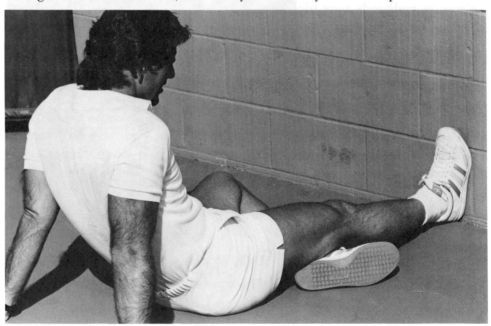

Isometrics for
the Achilles
tendon

When the pain is gone, do toe raises first on the floor and later on a step to increase the range of motion. After a week, add somewhat eccentric exercises such as uphill stair running. Ideally you should find a place with forty to fifty stairs and do them in sets to a level of comfortable fatigue. To make them more difficult, add a weight vest or belt. (Hand weights will not work because it is difficult to carry enough weight in the hands to effectively increase the resistance on the leg muscles, which are much stronger.) These exercises were designed primarily to build quad strength, but they also strengthen the ankle. Running up stairs is eccentric for the Achilles, but not as heavily so as in tennis, and therefore is a good transition exercise between injury and return to play. Finally, get back into play slowly over a seven- to ten-day period, starting with drills and progressively working into competitive play.

Tennis-related knee problems can take many forms. The sport's twisting, explosive motions can occasionally lead to a serious internal derangement of the knee, such as torn cartilage or ligaments. Patello-femoral joint pain, or pain related to the kneecap and knee joint, is also common. And sometimes knee problems are caused simply by overuse and the heavily eccentric muscle contractions involved in tennis.

Differentiating knee pains is a job for your sports medicine physician. Any problem that is recurrent or persists for more than a week should be investigated. Waiting too long for a knee pain to go away can have unfortunate results.

Concentric leg exercises on a stationary bicycle are a very effective way to strengthen the knee. They are suitable not only for prevention but also for the rehabilitation of, for example, torn cartilage or ligament problems. For an acutely symptomatic knee, however, it may be difficult to do even this exercise if the tension is too great. Instead, try riding the bike at a lower tension. Isometric wall-sit exercises can be substituted for or supplement the bicycle exercise. Bend your knees to a ninety-degree angle or as close to a ninety-degree angle as possible. Sit with your back facing against a wall in an imaginary chair. Hold this position for as long as you can, and repeat to a point of comfortable fatigue.

Despite the fact that it is widely prescribed, one apparatus that should be avoided is the knee extension machine. Unlike the leg press, it activates only the quadriceps and does not involve the hamstrings or upper calf muscles. When the quads are activated in this isolated manner, the rela-

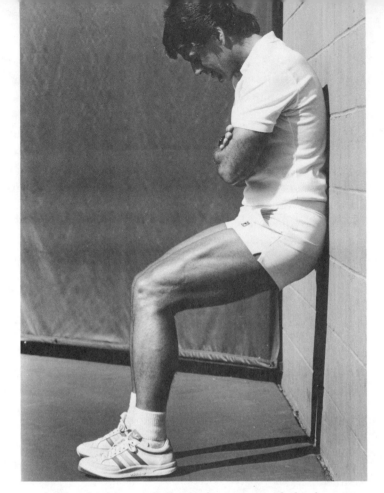

The isometric
wall-sit

tionship of the kneecap to the thighbone (femur) changes, and the kneecap
can grind against the condyles of the femur. Knee pain often results either
from abnormal strain on the patellar or quadriceps tendons, or from the
kneecaps grinding against the condyles of the femur. This does not happen
in the leg press, because the hamstrings and calf muscles are also activated
and hold the bones of the knee in their correct anatomical position.

Many therapists advocate knee extension exercises that put you through
only a limited part of the motion (usually the last thirty degrees before the
knee is completely straight). This certainly lessens the problem of the kneecap's grinding against the femur. It also means, however, that the quadriceps
can only develop about 30 to 40 percent of its maximum tension, so its
benefit as a knee-strengthening exercise is very limited.

While most injuries have nonsurgical solutions, some situations, particularly in the knee, may require early surgery. One patient of mine, an

executive with a major hotel corporation and a former collegiate tennis star, had knee problems including pain, consistent swelling after play, and occasional locking (when the joint momentarily sticks in one place) for a period of years. He put off doing something about his knee, because he thought he could work through the problem. When he finally did seek help, we first tried to build up his knee strength. After two months, he was stronger but the knee still swelled and throbbed. He then reluctantly agreed to surgery.

We ultimately removed many calcified lumps called loose bodies from his knees, as well as badly torn and frayed cartilage. Unfortunately, however, the problem had gone on for so many years that the loose bodies and torn cartilage had gouged the thighbone's joint surface. Since the surgery, he has had less pain, but his knee still occasionally swells and gives him trouble after a match. Had he attended to his knee years earlier, he most likely could have played with no pain whatsoever, because it is much easier to correct a little problem than a big one.

## Gearing Up

The burgeoning interest in tennis that began in the sixties sparked a revolution in the technology of the sport. Metal racquets, which were one of the first innovations, had actually been invented in the twenties by Rene Lacoste, among others. But it was Howard Head, the brilliant engineer-inventor who also introduced the first metal skis, who changed tennis with his Head Prince, a metal racquet with a very oversized head. At first, people regarded it more as a curiosity than a practical alternative, but today it and the other metal and composite racquets have become so popular that wooden racquets are now seldom seen on the courts anymore.

The shift has occurred because the wood racquets are less durable and harder to maneuver quickly. The metal or composite racquets have less wind resistance and can thus be moved faster, providing the theoretical advantage of more power.

Manufacturers often base their ad campaigns on this feature of the synthetic racquet. For most tennis players, however, the problem is not a lack of power but a lack of control. Because the wood racquet slows your swing down, it may actually be more suited to your needs. The best solution is to try a number of racquets and play with the one that feels best to you. If you haven't played before, enlist the aid of a USLTA (United States Lawn Tennis

Association) certified tennis professional in selecting a racquet.

I recommend beginning with a large-head racquet. It is easier to swing and enlarges the sweet spot, the part of the racquet from which the ball rebounds with the greatest energy. This enlarged sweet spot tends to make you hit the ball somewhat closer to the hand, which facilitates control.

Aluminum frames tend to be less expensive than other synthetic frames, and may be the best place to start. The Head Prince is still excellent, but many other manufacturers are making excellent large-frame, lightweight racquets. If possible, go to a shop that lets you try demonstrator racquets. Actually playing with the racquet will give you a much better feel for what works than will swinging them around in the store.

Strings are less of a problem now that racquets are no longer made primarily of wood. The best strings are catgut (really made from the gut of a lamb), but they are very expensive. Since the larger frames break strings more easily, consider the less costly and vastly improved synthetic strings, especially if you are just starting out.

The grip of the racquet is very important, because it determines in large part how your wrist will move when you hit the ball and therefore how much control you will have. A grip that is too small will tend to make your wrist flop around, which requires a degree of control found only in a few players. A larger grip makes it easier to hold the wrist more firmly. This generally is the preferred way to hit a tennis ball, and also is the form least likely to produce injuries.

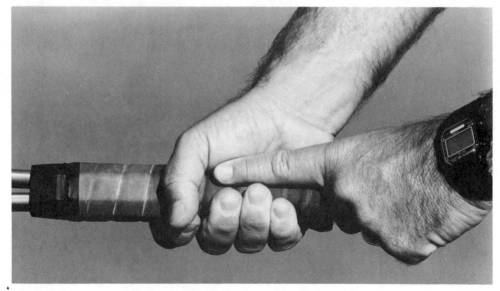

Getting the
right-size grip

To measure the grip, place the racquet handle in the palm of your hand and wrap your fingers around it. There should be about one finger width between the end of your fingers and the edge of your palm. If you can wrap your hand around the handle and touch your fingers to your palm, the grip is too small. Don't worry as much if the racquet is too small, because you can always build it up with tape. There is no way to compensate for a racquet handle that is too big, except by buying another racquet.

To cushion the foot from the shocks of sudden stop-starts, and provide lateral support for tennis' side to side moves, good shoes are vital. As with running shoes, don't be tempted to scrimp when buying them.

Some shoes are made primarily with a single court surface in mind, so be sure to take that into account when buying a pair. The Tretorn canvas-top shoe from Sweden, for example, is designed for clay courts, which are forgiving and soft. The shoe is wonderfully comfortable and useful for clay, but is inadequate for the hard courts most Americans play on. In general, leather-top or nylon-mesh shoes provide more stability than canvas top and are better for hard court surfaces.

The shoe must also be constructed with a good heel cushion that should be thicker under the heel than under the ball of the foot. This helps prevent excess strain on the Achilles tendon during the push-off motion as the player goes after the ball.

Take ten to fifteen minutes in the store to make sure the shoe is comfortable and fits well. You can break tennis shoes in, but the break-in period can be devastating to your feet.

## Tennis in STEP

Running stadium steps or hills for about thirty to forty yards until comfortable fatigue sets in will improve the explosive speed competitive tennis demands, and should be done as part of your STEP workout.

Working out three times a week for ten minutes at a time with the racquet itself is also useful. Put the racquet cover on and increase resistance by adding books inside the cover or wrapping the racquet head with lead tape. Some tennis shops now have special weights which attach to the strings, and are ideal for this exercise. Start with the forehand stroke and swing as if you were about to hit a forehand. Find the resistance (books or weights) that causes fatigue after about twenty to twenty-five times. If you can swing the racquet properly but for fewer times, lower the resistance. For those with weak wrists or arms or for those just beginning the game, the racquet cover will probably be about right. When the muscles fatigue, immediately do the isometric exercises. This will build strength in the muscles responsible for the forehand. Then do the same for the backhand, serve, and volley strokes.

While STEP is critical, one commonly performed exercise using ankle weights during the drill sessions should be avoided. It produces an abnormal stride and places new and unnecessary stresses on the lower extremities, especially the knees. You can increase resistance safely by wearing either a weight belt or a weighted vest. The extra weight around the torso will develop more strength and balance but will not affect running stride.

## The Workouts

Good professional instruction in stroke mechanics is essential for those intending to make tennis their primary sport. It is much more difficult to correct a problem stroke than to learn it properly in the first place. Take lessons in tandem with the following workouts, which will improve your aerobic base and your ability to move on court. The combination will dramatically improve your game.

To make tennis an excellent aerobic activity, all you need to do is adopt one rule: you are going to keep the ball in play no matter what. Also, to do the drills effectively, find a willing and, more importantly, an able partner. If you can, get access to a tennis ball machine, which can be a very effective tool in keeping your tennis workout aerobic, in addition to sharpening your skills.

Start your warm-up by easily jogging around the court for three to five minutes. Then rally easily with your partner, preferably from half court. Move back to the baseline over a ten-to-fifteen-minute period, gradually increasing the intensity and pace of the movements.

This is very different from the usual tennis warm-up, which consists of hitting the ball back and forth a few times before beginning play. Take the extra time, which will not only make you much less prone to injury but will make you far more likely to play better.

## The Maintenance Program

The core of the maintenance program is a series of drills that should be done three to five times a week. You don't have to do the whole series every time, but by the end of the week you should have spent at least some time doing each drill. In addition to the drills, you should run, cycle, swim, or weight train at least twice a week.

The first drill is a crosscourt drill, which is the bread-and-butter shot in tennis. It also holds the greatest margin for error since the court is longer diagonally and the net lower in the middle than on the sides. Start with both you and your partner having to hit the ball into each other's forehand court. So that the workout is more aerobic, the ball must be hit with your forehand, which forces you to return to center court each time you hit the ball. If you don't, your opponent will force you into using your backhand. After this drill is completed, repeat it, using only the backhand side.

To make the drill interesting, play games of ten points. A rally begins when the ball is hit over the net crosscourt three consecutive times. You lose a point if you fail to put the ball into the forehand court or fail to use your forehand. Once you begin this drill, you will realize how difficult it is to win by overpowering your opponent. Letting the other player make a mistake is a far more effective strategy. Keeping the ball in play longer, of course, also makes the workout more aerobic.

To make the shot and drill more effective, pretend that the net is twice as high as it really is. This will make you hit the ball over the net higher, and will result in your placing it deeper into your opponent's court. Hitting the ball deep is another winning trait in tennis.

When good players do this drill, it often takes them ten or even twenty hits apiece to make a point. During this time, they are constantly moving. If you are just beginning and cannot do the drill, rent time on a ball machine and do the drills against it. Since most beginners will not be able to keep the ball in play long enough, this also is the only way the workout will be aerobically demanding.

More-advanced players can add variations to the drill, by having one player hit crosscourt and the other down the line. Scoring is the same as with the straight forehand/backhand crosscourt drills. Start after hitting it over the net three times. You can make the drill even better by raising the net five to six inches higher with sticks. This will tend to keep the ball in play longer, because hitting driving or winning shots is very difficult when the net is so high. Do one forehand crosscourt, one backhand crosscourt, and two crosscourt/down-the-line drills.

Another variation has one player fixed on the forehand side, hitting the ball alternately crosscourt and down the line. The other person must return the ball every time to his partner who stands in that one position. This drill is similar to repeats in running, since one player rests while the other runs back and forth covering the whole court. This is an easier drill than the down-the-line crosscourt drill, because there is less chance of error with only one person running from side to side. Repeat the drill with the stationary player remaining on the backhand side of the court. Then switch roles. Play games of ten points on each side.

A more grueling exercise is the lob-volley drill. One player stands at the net, the other at the baseline. Using one-half the singles court measured longitudinally, the player on the baseline hits a low ball just over the net. The net player volleys the ball back to the baseline and then the baseline player returns with a lob that must be hit as an overhead shot. The play continues in this manner, with the baseline player alternating between lobs and low drives, and the net player alternating between hitting volleys and overheads.

This drill improves consistency and court movement, especially for the net player. It is relatively easy for the person on the baseline, but the person at the net must constantly move back and forth, which is very tiring. We used to call this drill "up and downs." Play for ten points twice, each player getting a turn at the net. Again, the idea of drill is not bashing winners but keeping the ball in play as long as possible.

There is another drill that uses the same baseline and net positions but requires more skill. It improves court quickness and balance and provides a tremendous workout. All balls should be hit at half speed. The baseline player stands in one position and hits drop shots just over the net, alternating from backhand to forehand, making the person at the net run from side to side to retrieve the ball. It can be performed so that the net player hits the ball to the same spot, giving the baseline player a rest, or from one corner to the next, giving the baseline player a workout too. Remember that the purpose of the drill is movement, not winning, and keep the ball at half speed. Play ten-point games in these drills as well.

Spending forty-five to sixty minutes three times a week in these drills will improve anyone's game and guarantee that the workout will be aerobic. You can alternate these drills with three to four days a week of matches that incorporate the drill's techniques and skills. Also, to help balance your body from the peculiarly one-sided stresses of tennis, I recommend three days a week of very easy jogging, swimming, circuit weight training, or cycling, for twenty to thirty minutes each time. In addition, do the trunk exercises three times a week, either at the end of match play or drills, or as part of one of the alternate workouts.

### Maintenance for intermediate and advanced players

**Day One**—Drills
**Day Two**—Tennis match (or lessons)
**Day Three**—Long, slow distance run, cycle, or swim, or circuit weight training
**Day Four**—Drills
**Day Five**—Tennis match (or lessons)
**Day Six**—Drills
**Day Seven**—Long, slow distance run, cycle, or swim, or circuit weight training

Novice or beginning players should follow the same schedule as the intermediate and advanced players, but do the drills with a ball machine to guarantee an effective workout.

## The Training Program

Before you can use the training program effectively, you will probably have to play seriously for at least one year. Work with a coach or teacher on the fine points of your strokes and use the workouts to prepare your body for the stress of increased play and competition, and for the extra strength, stamina, and speed necessary to win.

It will take years to get your skills to master levels, but training for peak physiological performance is the same in tennis as it is in other sports. From a good training base, it should take three months of intense drills and other exercises, performed in a pattern of alternating hard and easy days, to hone your skills and your physiological strength. For intervals, you are going to

need a coach or a ball machine. The drills can then be done in forty-five-
to sixty-second intervals and can use either side-to-side moves on a baseline,
or at the net doing volleys, or overhead and volley drills with the coach at
the baseline and you at the net. Then, after the work period, rest for thirty
seconds before starting again. Do these interval-type drills three times a
week during the intense training period.

Don't play matches on the days that you do these workouts; save them for
the other four days in the week. Instead, follow these interval workouts with
the trunk exercises.

On the four days that you play matches, finish the workout by swimming
or jogging at a low intensity for twenty to thirty minutes. This will help
correct muscular imbalances that result from the daily playing of the game.

The training workouts in this chapter are different from the programs in
the other sports because tennis requires a greater degree of nonendurance-
related skill. As a result, the principles of endurance training cannot be as
rigorously applied. The techniques outlined, however, will help you peak
physiologically and enter the tournament playing at the height of your ability.

In addition to lessons, then, the training workouts should be scheduled
as follows:

*Day One*—Match play plus swimming or running
*Day Two*—Drills plus trunk exercises
*Day Three*—Match play plus swimming or running
*Day Four*—Drills plus trunk exercises
*Day Five*—Match play plus swimming or running
*Day Six*—Drills plus trunk exercises
*Day Seven*—Match play plus swimming or running

## The Cool-Down

Finish each tennis workout with a series of stretches. If you do a post-tennis
swim or run, save your stretches until afterward.

## Racquetball

In the last ten years, racquetball has established itself as an alternative to
tennis and the second major racquet sport in America. One reason for its
popularity is economic—every aspect of the sport except for the shoes is

cheaper than tennis, including the balls, the racquet, the clubs, and the court time. Even the clothing is cheaper, since a T-shirt and gym shorts usually will suffice, as opposed to the designer apparel considered de rigueur for tennis. It is an indoor sport, so it is not dependent on the weather. Best of all, especially when compared to tennis, it doesn't take long to learn— most people can play a decent game within a few months.

These advantages notwithstanding, racquetball is not necessarily the tremendous aerobic sport its proponents claim. Elite racquetball players have about the same aerobic capacity that elite tennis players have, which means they still do not approach the levels of endurance of cross-country skiers, runners, cyclists, or swimmers. But although it may not be the ultimate aerobic exercise, it can still form the base of an aerobically effective exercise program.

This may take some work, however, because the game can and usually is played in a nonaerobic way. All the walls on the court are live, or in bounds, so the ball tends to come to the center of the room. It is possible, therefore, to move around the court surprisingly little and still hit the ball. Rather than wait and play to the center, however, a good player knows how to place the ball away from the center. This forces his opponent to run in order to retrieve the ball, and not only makes the game more challenging but more aerobic as well.

To help develop your ability and at the same time improve the aerobic benefits of the exercise, the *Athletics for Life* racquetball workouts incorporate two drills that teach you to place the ball with precision and give you speed. The first requires that both you and your opponent position yourself just behind the service line and in the center of the court. Hit the ball down one of the sidewalls as you would a serve, so that the ball bounces off the ceiling about three feet from the front wall and lands behind the service line but not off the back wall. Your opponent will then have to move from center court to retrieve the ball. He hits it off the ceiling in a similar manner, so that the ball lands behind the service line. Afterward, he returns to the starting position at center court.

This drill will be practiced on both sides of the court, so that you can hone both your forehand and your backhand ceiling shots. All balls must land between the service line and the back wall, and have to be hit with either the forehand or the backhand, depending on which side of the court the drill is taking place. The ball must land within the territory three times before a point is scored. After that third hit, a point is scored when one player fails to hit the ball so that it lands in the proper part of the court or fails to hit it with the proper stroke. Play games of ten on both sides of the court.

On the surface, this drill may appear to require very little movement. If you resist the temptation of going for a kill shot, however, you will be surprised at how much you have to move to do it right. Apart from making the workout more aerobic, this drill will teach you how to hit with precision and also get you used to maintaining optimal court position, which is one of the most important skills in winning.

In the second drill, the first player hits ceiling shots down the sidewalls. The second player retrieves the ball and hits toward the ceiling at approximately the center of the front wall, so that the ball bounces toward the other side of the court. In anticipation, the first player runs across the court, retrieves it, and hits it down the sidewall. The second player runs to the ball and again hits it to the center of the front wall, sending it back to the other side of the court. Score this drill the same way you did the first. After a game of ten points, switch positions.

This drill is more difficult than the first one for two reasons. First of all, you have to cover the entire court. Second, instead of concentrating exclusively on only one stroke, both players have to alternate between their forehands and their backhands.

To be more successful at the drill, move early. Most people tend to watch where the racquetball, or tennis ball, for that matter, goes and react only after the ball has effectively arrived at its destination. But good players anticipate the location of the ball and are moving toward that spot almost immediately. Since the location of the ball in these drills is known, anticipating its destination is much easier.

A second way to be more successful both in the drills and in your match play is to think only about where you are hitting the ball, not how you are going to hit it. In other words, imagine the spot on the front wall where you are going to hit to. As you make contact with the ball, think only about that spot, rather than about the specific biomechanical motion necessary to get it there. This skill is used unconsciously by all professional athletes, because it helps prevent you freezing up or becoming so preoccupied with things that you must do that you lose the fluid rhythm and instincts necessary for quick reactions.

If you are serious about the sport, there is also no substitute for professional instruction. Although racquetball can be mastered much more quickly than tennis, it is more a game of winners than tennis is, meaning that you get more points by winning placements than you do by unforced opponent errors. The most effective way to acquire these skills is through instruction and practice.

Racquetball has a relatively low incidence of injuries because the racquet and ball have a low mass. Tennis elbow is fairly common because of the tendency to lock the elbow rigidly before hitting a backhand, but is reported with a somewhat lower frequency than in tennis. In general, stresses on the arm and shoulder are also significantly less troublesome than in tennis. Low back and knee strains are a possible problem because of the low position required for kill shots. And, as with any sport that involves running, ankle sprains may also occur.

To treat or prevent these problems, refer to the section on tennis injuries earlier in this chapter. The biomechanics and motions of the two sports are very similar, as are the preventive remedies. Make sure, however, that you substitute a racquetball racquet for a tennis racquet in the arm and shoulder exercises.

Because racquetball started to gain popularity well after the technological revolution in tennis had begun, racquetball equipment was relatively sophisticated even in its early days. The equipment now is fairly standard, and is not that critical. Still, it is a good idea in any case to consult a racquetball professional about getting a racquet that is right for you. Finally, eye shields should be worn for protection from the ball.

## Racquetball in STEP

The serious player can sharpen his racquetball skills with a STEP workout. Like the exercise described in the tennis STEP workout, at the end of your game cover the racquet with its cover and weight it down with books, a one-pound sandbag, or lead tape. Then spend ten minutes going through the motions of the shots with this added resistance. Repeat each stroke as many times as it takes to fatigue the muscles. If you can do any stroke more than twenty-five times, add more resistance by increasing the weight of the racquet cover. Do this after the game because major strength gains are made when the muscles are already somewhat fatigued.

Long, slow distance running with periodic one hundred-meter sprints at 80 to 100 percent of your maximal effort will help train the muscles of your legs and arms for the quick motion necessary to the sport. Follow this with stair running, which is great for developing the explosive leg power racquetball demands. Begin the stair workouts by running at a moderate speed. Gradually build up to the point where you can bound up the stairs at full speed two and even three stairs at a time. As an alternative, go up two stairs at a time, but leap up them sideways so that you zig-zag. This prepares you for racquetball's lateral motions. If you are interested in maintaining your level of fitness, do these stair runs three times a week, working to a comfortable level of fatigue each time.

Circuit resistance training, with the emphasis on conditioning rather than strength gains, can also help your game. Swimming and cycling can be used as well, as they are nongravity sports that provide variety and build a good aerobic base.

## The Workouts

The serious racquetball player will probably want to play the game every day, despite the benefits of a more varied fitness program. Casual players are more likely to be satisfied with three to five games a week, and can therefore get the benefits of training with other sports as well. Regardless of which camp you fall into, perform the drills at least three times a week, following them with a rigorous game of match play.

## The Maintenance Program for the Casual Player

*Day One*—Drills plus game

*Day Two*—Long, slow distance workout in sport of choice

*Day Three*—Drills plus game

*Day Four*—Long, slow distance workout in sport of choice plus circuit weight training

*Day Five*—Drills plus game

*Day Six*—Long, slow distance workout in sport of choice plus circuit weight training

*Day Seven*—Rest or match play

## The Maintenance Program for the Serious Player

This program isn't easy, but it will provide the physical base that will send you into any tournament without being able to use your physical condition as an excuse for playing badly.

*Day One*—Drills plus game plus STEP
*Day Two*—Long, slow distance run, cycle, or swim plus circuit resistance exercises
*Day Three*—Drills plus game plus STEP
*Day Four*—Drills plus game plus STEP
*Day Five*—Long, slow distance run, cycle, or swim plus circuit resistance exercises
*Day Six*—Drills plus game plus STEP
*Day Seven*—Match play

## The Training Program

To peak for a certain tournament or event, you have to make still other additions. Increased court time and match play are essential, as is playing with a coach who can teach you the proper strategy and refine your technique.

With respect to peaking physically, continue your stair or hill running. But instead of working to comfortable fatigue, work to maximum fatigue twice a week. Follow the stair or hill running by going onto a football field that is not being used and running side to side between the goal posts, which have the same dimensions as a racquetball court. Pretend to hit a forehand as you arrive at one end of the goal post and a backhand as you sprint back to the other. Do this ten times, rest for one minute; do another set of ten, rest for a minute; and then do a final set of ten.

It may seem unnecessary to do this on a football field instead of a court, but try it a few times. I find that it is often better to perform these exhaustive workouts off the court, so that the court itself doesn't become associated with drudgery and can be approached with vigor and excitement.

As in peaking with other sports, begin training three months prior to the event. Follow this training schedule:

**Day One**—Racquetball match play plus weighted racquet STEP exercise

**Day Two**—Drills with coach in the morning; stair or hill running and football field running in the afternoon or evening

**Day Three**—Racquetball match play plus weighted racquet STEP exercises

**Day Four**—Drills with coach in the morning; stairs or hill running and football field running in the afternoon or evening

**Day Five**—Racquetball match play plus weighted racquet STEP exercise

**Day Six**—Drills with coach in the morning; stair or hill running in the afternoon

**Day Seven**—Match play

## The Cool-Down

Finish each workout with a series of stretches described on pp. 187–94.

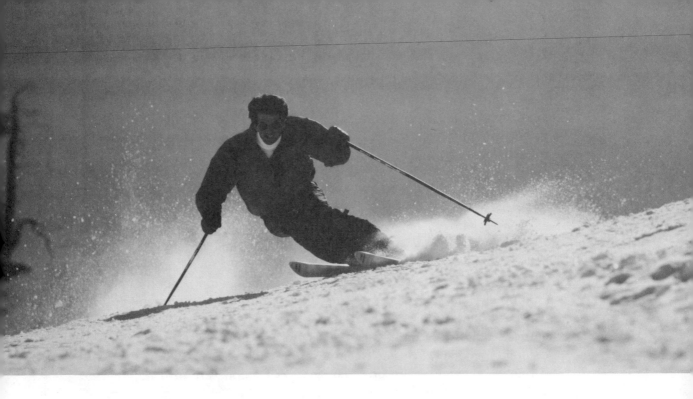

## Cross-Country (Nordic) Skiing

IKE many people who grew up on alpine, or downhill, skiing, I approached cross-country skiing with a condescending attitude. I had done some cross-country skiing from time to time over the years, but never out of a conscious choice. I knew, of course, of cross country's tremendous physiological benefits. In fact, because it involves more of the body's muscles simultaneously than any other activity, it is the best aerobic activity available. But its being vigorous exercise was virtually the only impression I had of the sport.

I probably would never have become a true convert had not one of my best friends, John Slouber, who himself had been an alpine ski racer, opened a cross-country ski resort. Several winters ago, he invited me to participate

Skiing 7

in his first "California Gold Rush," a by-now famous fifty-five-kilometer cross-country marathon that has become the championship event of the Great American Ski Chase. Since we hadn't seen each other in a long time and I am always ready for a competitive event, I decided the race was a good excuse for us to get together.

To my surprise, I actually enjoyed the skiing and began to appreciate the level of skill the sport requires. I remember watching the American and Scandinavian ski teams warming up before the start of the first race, and being surprised by the speed they could attain and the grace they exhibited. As I later tried (none too successfully at first) to emulate their skill, I realized I had shortchanged cross-country skiing.

Until a few years ago, cross-country skiing consisted of stopping the car, strapping on your skis, and traipsing through the woods. This may be fun, but it lacks the exhilaration of skiing on beautifully manicured trails. Now that these trails are becoming the norm at cross-country ski resorts throughout the country, the sport is much more exciting and accessible.

Dramatic refinements in cross-country ski fashions are also helping the sport's image. Not long ago, a typical cross-country ski outfit consisted of baggy pants, a down-filled parka, and mittens. Today, however, tight-fitting Lycra racing suits, brightly colored sweaters, ski tights, and a host of other accoutrements make Nordic skiwear every bit as colorful and flattering as that found on downhill slopes.

Changes in equipment have also helped upgrade not just the sport's image but also the ease with which you can ski. Until about five years ago, skiers generally used wooden skis, whose bases required careful preparation, including an application of wax geared to the day's snow conditions. Today's composite skis have plastic bases that don't need to be waxed, making it possible to get on the trails without any fuss or guesswork.

With the advent of roller skis, especially the newer, safer ones, even winter is no longer a prerequisite. With them, you can practice the sport's movements even in the summer. Champion skiers, in fact, may spend almost as much time on their rollers as they do their regular skis.

Cross-country skiing is also an affordable sport, usually costing one-third to one-half less than downhill skiing. Equally important, it is a very safe sport. In alpine skiing, the foot is firmly fixed to the ski, but in cross-country skiing, only the toe is strapped into the ski. The rest of the foot retains a considerable degree of motion, even in a fall. This flexibility results in far fewer ankle and knee sprains than in downhill skiing.

All in all, then, cross-country skiing is highly recommended to anyone interested in fitness and or in learning a new skill sport (including devout alpine skiers like myself who insist that cross-country skiing has nothing to offer them). It is certainly great for people in colder climates who previously brought their fitness programs indoors or gave them up for the winter. Thanks to roller skis, it can even be a year-round activity.

## The Safety Factor

Even though cross-country skiing is relatively safe, you can sprain your ankle, knee, or thumb in a fall. For these injuries, follow the advice given for almost any athletic injury, summarized by the acronym RICE (rest, ice, compression, and elevation).

Assume, for example, that you fall and twist your ankle. If continued motion is painful, enlist the aid of a friend or the ski patrol and go to the nearest shelter. Once there, fill a garbage bag with snow or ice, lie down on a couch, and elevate your leg with one or more cushions. If an Ace bandage is available, wrap it around your foot. Start at the toe and make continuous overlapping circles with the bandage to the top of your calf. Then ice the ankle.

These measures will minimize the swelling or inflammation caused by the fall. Though a natural body response to the injury, swelling ultimately slows down the healing process. Try to apply these measures within thirty minutes after the injury, because the sooner they are applied, the more effective they will be. Rest, ice, compression, and elevation are still appropriate in the forty-eight hours after the injury, but the first thirty minutes are the most important.

Some falls, of course, are truly minor. Causing only momentary discomfort, they won't prevent you from continuing the activity. Other falls are more insidious. If you can't continue skiing right after the fall but feel better the next morning, resist the temptation to resume the activity with full vigor, The R in RICE means rest, and is included in the prescription because apparently minor injuries of this kind are susceptible to more inflammation and further injury. A limp or pain means you should take the day off and, if possible, see a physician, because the injury may be more severe than you think. If you decide you are able to ski, use the 75/75 rule—ski only terrain that is 75 percent as difficult as you normally ski, and ski at only 75 percent of your normal intensity.

Overuse aches and pains are more common in cross-country skiing than injuries. The two areas where you are most likely to feel these aches, especially on your first attempts, are the low back and the back of the upper arms and shoulders. You might expect the legs to be the first to feel the stress, but the leg motion in cross-country skiing is more concentric and therefore, like cycling, quite forgiving. The trunk motion, on the other hand, requires a forward lean with each stride that makes the exercise eccentric for the low back muscles and thus more likely to provoke muscle soreness. The arms get sore because they are vigorously used for propulsion and, depending on the skill level, for balance. The balancing aspect of pole activity is heavily eccentric as well. The best way to treat these problems is preventively, through the STEP exercise described on page 139.

The biggest potential danger in cross-country skiing comes not from the sport itself but from the environment and the possibility of hypothermia. Hypothermia, which is the reduction of the core body temperature to below ninety-five degrees Fahrenheit, can actually occur in all kinds of weather, not just in winter. In fact, there are numerous fatal cases of hypothermia reported each summer in seventy-degree weather in places like the High Sierras. Cold weather, however, accentuates the danger.

Hypothermia is caused by losing too much body heat. When you are active, a by-product of muscle metabolism is heat energy. The body radiates this heat out into the environment. The more work you do, the more heat you radiate. While some heat loss is necessary, too much heat loss is dangerous.

The chain of events leading to hypothermia in summertime hikers begins, for example, with the lightly clad hiker exerting himself and rapidly dispersing heat from his body. Because of the higher altitude, his breathing rate is substantially increased. There is a good deal of water vapor in the exhaled air, so this increased breathing rate results in a dramatic loss of fluid. Unless this fluid is replaced, the body's core temperature begins to increase. The body tries to lose this heat by shunting blood to the skin and dilating the blood vessels. When the blood circulates near the skin, heat is radiated out to the environment. A situation that begins as hyperthermia, or excess body heat, can actually switch and become hypothermia, with one of the key factors being the level of hydration.

Although wearing more clothes than the hiker, a cross-country skier can go through the same process. Cross-country skiing requires a great deal of exertion and is accompanied by increased breathing. This results in a substantial loss of fluid and, despite the winter temperatures, an increase in the core body temperature. Blood is shunted to the skin and radiates heat into the environment. If too much heat is lost, hypothermia occurs.

Prevention is the best medicine. Although you cannot regulate the outside temperature, you can control the amount and intensity of your workout, the preservation of body heat through appropriate clothing, and the replacement of lost fluid.

To conserve heat, protect your head, abdomen, and thorax, which radiate the greatest amount of heat, by wearing layers of clothes. Next to the body, choose garments made of cotton, which wicks moisture from the skin, rather than nylon. Wear a lightweight or heavy wool sweater over them. For extra protection, wear a down vest or a lightweight windbreaker as a final outer layer. And don't forget to wear a warm hat.

Fluids can also help prevent hypothermia, because they are instrumental in the body's maintenance of a more normal central core temperature. It is possible, for example, for a one hundred sixty-pound cross-country skier to lose three to four liters per hour. Even in moderate workouts, fluid losses of one to two liters an hour are possible.

The best way to replace the lost fluids during vigorous exercise is to drink a dilute sugar solution containing 2–4 percent carbohydrates and 98–96 percent water throughout the exercise. This allows for the replacement of some calories, so that the muscles do not become depleted of their glycogen supplies. More important, keeping the solution dilute ensures that as much fluid as possible will be absorbed from the stomach. When more concentrated carbohydrate solutions are present in the stomach, it empties much more slowly. When fluid replacement is vitally important, keeping the fluids dilute is critical.

Several companies now manufacture "sports" drinks that are supposed to replace the lost fluids, but most are overly concentrated. Look on the carton of such drinks for the number of grams of carbohydrates per serving. The ideal drink should have from twenty-five to forty grams of carbohydrates per liter (one thousand milliliters of fluid), which would make it a 2½–4 percent carbohydrate solution.

Regardless of the amount of fluid lost, the body can absorb only a certain amount of liquid in a given time, even if the fluid is plain water. That means you must replace lost fluid regularly.

Don't rely on thirst as a signal of whether or not you are properly hydrated. Physiological investigations of people exercising in heat has shown that the thirst mechanism shuts off at relatively low levels of exercise. We don't know why this happens, but we see its dangerous side effects all too often after endurance races such as triathlons and marathons.

Rather than wait until you are thirsty, then, you must drink fluids regularly when exercising strenuously. Although the amount will vary from individual to individual, a one hundred sixty-pound skier, for example, should drink about one cup of liquid every fifteen minutes. People who weigh less should drink proportionately less, and people who weigh more should drink proportionately more.

One of the most dangerous aspects of hypothermia is its insidious onset. Lethal vital organ damage occurs at about 85 degrees Fahrenheit, but other symptoms are present long before the damage is irreversible. The first stages of the condition, however, often are not evident to the victim or even to the people around him. Among the key symptoms are a generalized feeling of lassitude, indifference, and fatigue. Sometimes an afflicted person will simply sit down and allow the rest of the group to go on without him. Should such a situation occur, get the person out of the wind and cold and give him fluids or food. If the person is only tired, he will feel better in several minutes. Someone suffering from hypothermia will stay the same or deteriorate unless measures are taken. Do whatever you can to increase his temperature. If you are skiing with a group, ask another skier to notify the ski patrol. Never leave someone in this condition alone.

Unless you are skiing a circuit in which you are never more than a few minutes away from a warming hut or lodge, it is foolish to ski without a fanny pack. More often than not, you will be miles away from warmth, food, and shelter, and should be able to provide each in the event of an emergency.

For warmth, put a thermal, aluminum-foil-type blanket in your kit. It weighs only a few ounces, but when wrapped around you can be a lifesaver because it prevents you from radiating heat from the body. Even the smallest amount of wind exposure will greatly increase the rate of heat loss, so do whatever you can to get out of the wind. If you are near a tree, take shelter behind it. Try to break off a few boughs so that you don't have to sit on the snow, and put the thermal blanket around you. If no trees are available, use your skis and poles to carve a hole in the snow big enough for you to fit in. By reducing your exposure to the wind, you reduce subsequent heat loss.

For nourishment, carry some densely caloric food in your pack. Candy bars or other fatty foods are excellent for these emergency situations, because there are two times the amount of calories in a gram of fat than in a gram of sugar or protein. Since you will not be moving, fluid losses will not be a major concern. Use thirst as your guide and eat small amounts of snow to maintain hydration.

While hypothermia can happen anywhere, frostbite is a problem only in colder climates. It is much more likely when wind and cold exposure occur at the same time. The most commonly afflicted areas are the toes, fingers, ears, tip of the nose, cheeks, and chin. The simplest remedy and prevention is wearing some protection against the wind and staying out of subzero temperatures. In Scandinavia, all ski competitions are stopped when the temperature drops to zero degrees Fahrenheit, because even the wind the skier creates at this temperature can cause frostbite.

Most cases of "frostbite" are actually frostnip, and result in no permanent damage. Although it can happen quickly, frostbite usually results only when there has been prolonged exposure to wind and cold. In the past, frostbite used to be treated by amputation. Interestingly, surgeons experienced with this problem have now learned that the body will auto-amputate the dead tissues to the most appropriate degree. This tends to preserve more viable tissue than surgical amputation, which usually removes more tissue than is necessary.

Lastly, don't forget to take special precautions to protect your eyes. Snow blindness occurs when the sun's radiation burns the cornea, which has a high concentration of nerves. I know from personal experience that this can be a very painful condition. I never liked wearing sunglasses, and often skied during late spring without eye protection. One year, I finally suffered snow blindness. In addition to being in acute pain for about a week, I am now permanently sensitized to the sun to the point that even minor exposure without sunglasses is painful.

Sunburn can also be a problem because you are exposed to more solar radiation in the snow and mountains than at any other time, including when you are on the ocean. Everyone, regardless of skin coloration or ease of tanning, should wear a sunscreen. It must have PABA or one of its newer analogues, which have the proven ability to filter harmful solar rays.

To protect yourself, apply a sunscreen at least thirty minutes before going out in the sun. The active ingredient in the sunscreen takes at least that long to bond with the skin. If you go out before it does, you can burn before the sunscreen's protective qualities take effect.

## Equipment

For the last five years, there has been an almost complete revolution in cross-country ski technology. The boot-binding interface, for example, has changed dramatically. Before, leather boots and a binding of pins that went through the front of the sole of the shoe were the rule. There was very little torsional rigidity in these leather soles, so controlling the ski was difficult. Boots today are made from plastics, which offer a great deal of rigidity and thus make control of the ski much easier.

Some boot manufacturers now make boot-binding systems so that selecting the right boot and binding is much easier than it was. Before buying, read the yearly equipment guide in *Cross Country Skier*.

Cross-country skis have also benefited from the technological revolution. Only a short time ago, all skis were made out of wood and were more or less the same. Today, almost all are synthetic composites. Lightweight, they have tremendously improved gliding properties, and can also be precision manufactured for a broad range of abilities. An elite racer's stiff skis, for instance, would be completely unsuitable for a beginner, who needs wider, more flexible, and more easily manuevered skis.

As important as the changes in the skis themselves are the changes that have taken place in the base or running surface of the skis. This is of primary importance to the beginner, because the newer waxless skis have remarkably good gliding qualities while still allowing good grip of the snow for a "kick." This was always the double dilemma of waxless skis: when they provided enough grip, the gliding was horrible, and vice versa. A measure of just how far the technology has come is that many international races are now won using waxless skis.

Ski length and stiffness are also important. A good length for the beginner or intermediate skier is a ski which comes to the wrist as you stand up and hold your hands straight above your head. Advanced skiers may prefer a little more length. To test stiffness, hold the skis together bottom to bottom. You should be able to hold and squeeze them together with the thumbs and two fingers of each hand. If you can't, they are too stiff, particularly if you are a beginner.

As previously noted, the bindings are dictated by the sole of the shoe you buy. Once you pick a shoe with the necessary lateral support and torsional rigidity, you have in effect determined the type of bindings you will use.

To select the right size poles, stand up and drop your arms to your side. The pole should reach halfway between the bottom of your armpit and the top of your shoulder. Some people prefer shorter poles, but with poling becoming increasingly important in the sport, the larger poles provide an advantage. Also, buy poles made of the newer, lightweight synthetic materials rather than the more old-fashioned bamboo.

The technology has progressed to the point where the industry is now entering a period of revision rather than revolution. Don't put off buying equipment for fear of its becoming immediately obsolete, because this is not likely to happen. On the other hand, the costs of a complete outfit are not insignificant, so renting your equipment from a cross-country specialty store or resort is an attractive option, especially if you are new to the sport.

## Cross-Country Skiing in STEP

The easiest way to do the STEP arm exercises is with wall pulleys, which provide you with a means of practicing almost the identical motions used in poling. The arms can be used individually, simulating the poling motions of diagonal striding, or simultaneously, to practice double poling. To condition the muscles, find a weight that allows you to continue the exercise for five minutes at the beginning stages of your training program. Work up to ten or even fifteen minutes of continuous poling by the end of the training program. When concentrating on strength, find a weight that allows you to do the poling motion about twenty-five times for each arm. When you are able to do twenty-five easily, increase the weight. Like other STEP exercises, this should be performed at least two and preferably three times a week.

## The Workouts

Because cross-country skiing is a seasonal sport, there are two sets of workouts, one for the off-season and one for the ski season.

### The off-season

The best way to prepare for the ski season is with long, slow distance running and cycling workouts. In tandem, they will improve your aerobic base and strengthen your legs. Use STEP to build up the upper body, and include the rowing machine, bar dips, and a slant board or wall pulleys that simulate the poling motion. Uphill or stair running will further develop leg strength and also prepare you for the terrain changes of skiing.

Advanced cross-country skiers now use a skating motion, so you should also do one workout a week either on roller skates to practice it. You may use them either at the end of a workout, or substitute roller skating or skiing for a long, slow distance running workout.

The maintenance program should be scheduled as follows:

> **Day One**—Long, slow distance running for forty-five to sixty minutes at 65 to 75 percent of the maximal heart rate
>
> **Day Two**—Long, slow distance cycling or running for forty-five to sixty minutes, followed by a STEP workout
>
> **Day Three**—Long, slow distance running workout
>
> **Day Four**—Long, slow distance workout on stationary bike, followed by STEP or circuit resistive exercises (see Chapter 9)
>
> **Day Five**—Long, slow distance running or speedplay running workout
>
> **Day Six**—Long, slow distance cycling or running workout, followed by STEP
>
> **Day Seven**—Long, slow distance roller skating, roller skiing, or ice-skating workout

### The ski season

With the ski season in full force, you need only do the STEP exercises if you feel they are necessary.

Schedule your workouts as follows:

> **Day One**—Long, slow distance cross-country skiing with optional STEP workout

**Day Two**—Long, slow distance cross-country skiing

**Day Three**—Long, slow distance swimming or stationary bicycle workout, followed by circuit resistive exercises

**Day Four**—Long, slow distance cross-country skiing

**Day Five**—Long, slow distance stationary bicycle or swimming workout, followed by circuit resistive exercises

**Day Six**—Modified speedplay cross-country ski workout

**Day Seven**—Long, slow distance cross-country skiing

## The Training Program

There are more and more cross-country races you can have fun with and train for every year. The finishing times closely parallel those of comparable distance running races, which means that the training programs of the two sports are similar. The major difference is in the STEP exercises.

Schedule the training workout for the first two weeks as follows:

**Day One**—Long, slow-distance cross-country ski workout

**Day Two**—Speedplay cross-country ski workout

**Day Three**—Long, slow-distance cross-country ski workout

**Day Four**—Speedplay cross-country ski workout

**Day Five**—Long, slow-distance cycling or swimming workout

**Day Six**—Speedplay cross-country ski workout

**Day Seven**—Long, slow-distance cross-country ski workout

Use these guidelines for weeks three through ten:

**Day One**—Long, slow distance cross-country ski workout

**Day Two**—Thirty minutes of easy skiing, followed by intervals

**Day Three**—Long, slow distance cycling workout

**Day Four**—Thirty minutes of easy skiing, followed by repeats

**Day Five**—Long, slow distance ski workout

**Day Six**—Thirty minutes of easy skiing, followed by intervals

**Day Seven**—Long, slow distance cycling workout

For week eleven, alternate one interval and two repeat workouts with four long, slow distance workouts, at least one of which is a cycling workout.

If you are carbo-loading on the twelfth week, use the following schedule:

*Day One*—Two-hour ski session at moderate intensity
*Day Two*—Thirty minutes of easy skiing
*Day Three*—Thirty minutes of easy skiing
*Day Four*—Thirty minutes of easy skiing, followed by optional moderate repeats
*Day Five*—Thirty minutes of easy skiing
*Day Six*—Thirty minutes of easy skiing
*Day Seven*—Rest

If you are not carbo-loading, use this schedule for week twelve:

*Day One*—Long, slow distance ski workout
*Day Two*—Long, slow distance cycling workout
*Day Three*—Thirty minutes easy skiing, followed by repeats
*Day Four*—Long, slow distance ski workout
*Day Five*—Long, slow distance cycling workout
*Day Six*—Thirty minutes easy skiing, followed by repeats
*Day Seven*—Rest

## The Cool-Down

Finish the workout with five to ten minutes of easy skiing and the appropriate stretches from pages 187–94.

## Alpine (Downhill) Skiing

When I was skiing internationally and training very hard, I frequently encountered the attitude that training for alpine skiing was unnecessary. "Why are you putting yourself through so much?" people would typically ask. "After all, you glide downhill and let gravity do all the work, so why make such a fuss?"

This attitude may well explain why downhill skiing is the most inherently dangerous sport we consider in this book. People underestimate its demands, and fail to realize that elite competitive alpine skiers have greater leg strength relative to their body weight than athletes of any other sports, and have aerobic powers that approach those of elite swimmers. This is a good indication that skiing is very demanding indeed.

Unfortunately, however, many casual skiers give little thought to their leg strength or aerobic power, and head out to the slopes with little or no preparation. Without adequate strength or conditioning, the falls inevitable to skiing are even more likely to occur.

Even if you ski only one week a year, you will benefit from the workouts in this part of the chapter, because they will send you to the slopes a well-prepared skier. By spending several months anticipating skiing's demands, you will be a less tired, a less injury-prone, and, most importantly, a better skier.

## Adjusting to the Altitude

One of the first problems skiers have is adjusting to the higher elevations. Often, we may not even recognize what is happening. Typically, we get to the resort, ski hard the first few days, and are exhausted by the third or fourth day. We blame the exhaustion on the activity itself, and fail to appreciate that much of the fatigue is caused by the high altitudes.

But at six thousand-feet elevation, which is the lowest point of almost all major ski resorts, there is significantly less oxygen in the air compared to sea level. To compensate and keep up with the body's demands for oxygen, the heart beats faster and the lungs breathe more frequently. Add this to the aerobic demands for oxygen from the activity itself, and you can see why you get tired, especially in the first few days at a ski resort.

Adaptation to high altitude actually takes place over many months, but about 80 percent of the critical adaptations involving the heart and lungs are made in the first four or five days—at precisely the point where most ski trips are winding down. Unfortunately, there is nothing you can do to minimize the amount of time it takes to adjust to the altitude. You *can* minimize the effects of the altitude and the extent of fatigue, however, by developing a good aerobic base and adequate strength before you get to the mountains.

## Equipment

There are so many factors to consider when you select equipment, including how often you ski, how well you ski, and what kind of snow you like, that a complete discussion of what to buy would be too extensive for the scope of this book. The skiing magazines cover the newest advances and products very well, and many of the ski shops can also be very helpful. If you are just beginning to ski or don't ski very often, rent your skis from a reputable ski shop. Rental skis are often superb, and don't have to be transported, stored, or maintained by you. They will also give you an idea of what kind of ski you like before you buy a pair.

Whether you rent or buy, you have to decide how long your skis will be. In the seventies, the tendency was toward short or even supershort skis. If you are a beginner, starting with these shorter skis can give you an early confidence because they are much easier to turn. However, I strongly recommend graduating to the longer skis as you improve. Don't be frightened of them; you will find that turning them is not as difficult as you probably imagined and that the added control they provide makes skiing on them like driving a Porsche after you have been used to an old Volkswagen.

A one hundred sixty-five-pound skier who is about five feet eleven, for example, might start on a 170–180 centimeter ski. As his ability progresses, he should move up to a longer ski, typically 200–210 centimeters for recreational skiing. Taller or shorter people should start with proportionately longer or shorter skis.

Even if you rent skis, consider buying your own ski boots. Unlike the boots of the past, today's ski boots should feel comfortable from the start. When you put the boot on, your foot shouldn't be able to move around. The heel should be snug but comfortable, and you should be able to move your toes without them feeling either lost or cramped. Try the boots out in the later afternoon, because any impediments to a normal fit, including swollen feet, will be more appreciable then. To avoid making a mistake, spend at least thirty minutes in the boots before buying them.

The most important requirement for poles is that they not be too long. To make sure yours are the right length, turn one upside down with its handle on the floor. Grasp the pole under the basket. Your forearm will be almost horizontal with the ground if the pole is the right height. The length of the poles is less important than the technique with which you use them, so consider taking lessons to learn the right form.

To be comfortable during the day, layer your clothes the same way a cross-country skier would.

## Alpine Skiing in STEP

Skiing injuries usually take two forms. The first are the sprains, fractures, contusions, and lacerations that result from a fall. Typically, you arrive at the ski slopes after months of anticipation and spend the first few days in an exhilarating burst of activity. By the third day, your body is fatigued and becomes much more susceptible to injury. Because of the fatigue, a fall that might be of little consequence on the first day can result on day three in serious injury. To make matters worse, fatigue leads to a greater likelihood of falling. You can exert little control over these injuries once they occur, but by being fitter and maintaining your equipment, the chances of these accidents are lowered considerably.

A second group of injuries includes the aches and pains that come from overuse. The third-day muscle soreness of the legs, lower back, and upper arms typically encountered by recreational skiers on their annual ski trips is essentially overuse injury, because the body takes from forty-eight to seventy-two hours to fully respond to the effects of eccentric exercise.

And skiing is a very eccentric exercise, especially for the lower back and quadriceps muscles. At the end of a turn, centrifugal force tries to make the body go down the hill. A good skier compensates for this force in part by sinking down and bending the knees and torso as the turn progresses. Thus, while the muscles are tightening, they are also being elongated by the bend, making the motion eccentric.

To mitigate against the possibility of injury, you should follow the pre-season workouts in this chapter, which make extensive use of STEP to strengthen each of the involved muscle groups. The ankle, for instance, used to be the most commonly injured body part in skiing. Now, however, boots encase the ankle and extend up the leg to the mid-calf, alleviating many, but not all, ankle injuries. In its place, the knee has become the most commonly injured part of the body. The best way to prevent these injuries is by properly preparing the musculature for the stress of skiing.

If you have strong knees and ankles, the tissues can withstand the force of a fall much more easily. To strengthen them, do the wall-sit and the penguin walk (see p. 113). The penguin walk should be done for one to four minutes before you stretch at the end of every running workout. Start slowly, gradually working up to four minutes for several weeks before you go skiing.

The wall-sit, which strengthens the quadriceps, should also be done at the end of the workout. Concentrate your weight on your heels and keep the knees at an angle of about ninety degrees. As with any other isometric exercise, exert as much force as you can. Start with thirty-second wall-sits, and work up to four minutes. By the time you can sit pressing hard against the wall for four minutes, you will be ready for almost any hill. Note that there is a big difference between simply maintaining the wall-sit position and actively pressing back against the wall. To do it right, you have to press against the wall.

To develop tolerance for the twisting forces of the turn, put your skis on the floor. With your ski boots on, sit on a stool and get into your skis. Bend the legs at ninety degrees and twist your feet as hard as you can in one

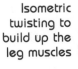

Isometric twisting to build up the leg muscles

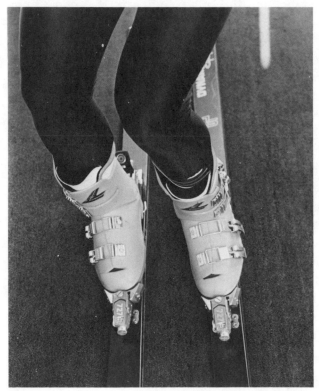

direction. Hold it for at least thirty seconds, and then twist your feet the other way. This exercise is particularly good because it prepares the knee for the slow twist, which is the most dangerous movement in skiing. When you twist on the snow, the skis will turn. On the carpet or floor, however, they won't move. The exercise thus becomes isometric. Placing more weight on the "outside" ski in your imaginary turn enables you to practice body angulation and correct pole position as well.

Hill running is another important STEP exercise that you should begin at least one, and preferably two, months before the ski season. Spring up a hill or stairs to develop the concentric leg strength necessary to push off the mountain and to turn; run down hills or stairs to prepare your legs for the eccentric motions. To avoid undue soreness or even injury, gradually ease into the downhill or downstairs running. Walking down them is probably a good idea for the first week or so of the program.

A trail that goes through a hilly or mountainous area and that has periodic ups and downs makes this exercise the most fun. If that is unavailable, any hill that is one hundred to two hundred meters long will work. If you are

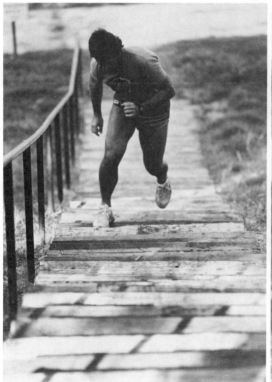 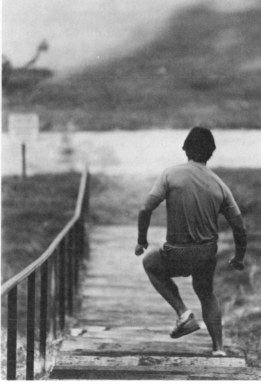

Uphill stair running (STEP)

Downhill stair running (STEP)

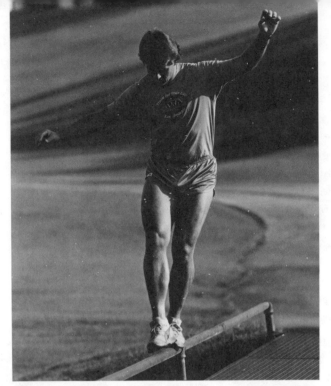

running down stairs, remember to guard against ankle sprains and falls. Though it is a great way to develop the specific strength and agility required in skiing, begin slowly until your confidence and skill are increased.

Do one of these STEP workouts a week for the first two weeks, two for the third and fourth weeks, and three per week for the second month. One day concentrate on the uphill portion, resting on the way down, and the next on the opposite direction. During downhill runs on a road or on grass, make turns every ten to twenty feet, so that you run down in an S pattern. When going up the hill, just run straight up. Start by running up and down the hill or stairs for ten to fifteen minutes. When you can work up to more than twenty-five to thirty minutes of hill work, you will be in very good shape indeed.

To develop balance, get a one-inch rope and stretch it tight between two trees from one to three feet off the ground. Then practice rope walking. Although you will probably fall frequently at first, there is nothing like rope walking to produce balance. With practice, you will be able to do exercises like squats or even one-leg, deep knee bends on the rope.

Other balancing exercises can be done on a wooden bar, such as a two-by-four placed flat on the floor. A bongo board (an eighteen-inch-long board with a round roller at its center that rolls back and forth) is also good. Even walking on railroad tracks—making sure beforehand that there are no trains—can enhance balance. Do at least one of these balancing exercises for five minutes each day.

The trunk is often overlooked in ski preparations. The exercises described in the tennis section will be effective here as well. To produce significant gains, perform them three times a week.

In competition and, to a lesser extent, recreational skiing, the arms and shoulder muscles are important. One of the best pieces of apparatus to develop them are wall pulleys on which the poling motion can be practiced. Select a weight you can do no more than twenty times and attempt to do three sets of twenty reps with the weight. If you can do the exercise more than twenty times, increase the resistance.

## The Off-Season

Follow the running program, performing STEP workouts on days two, four, and six after the running workout.

## The Ski Season

The maintenance ski program will keep the sport aerobic. To do that, the first rule, regardless of your skiing ability, is to ski the run from top to bottom, continually turning without stopping.

This is a big change from the way most recreational skiers stop and start and tend to track in long, straight lines between turns. To improve your skiing, don't do any straight running between the turns. Sometimes you will do long radius turns and build up faster speeds, and sometimes much shorter turns during which the speed is more controlled. In skiing, it is turning that controls speed; probably the biggest single mistake skiers make is failing to complete turns or not turning at all.

To ski this way, you will have to pay attention to the slopes that you ski on. If you are a beginner, you can't hope to ski proficiently on intermediate or advanced slopes. Instead, practice your technique on the beginner slopes until you are expert on them. Then move on to a more difficult run and repeat it until you become proficient on that one as well. This is different from the perception many people have of becoming an expert. They think that skiing on the harder slopes makes them improve, but it doesn't. All it does is increase your risk of injury and prevents you from improving more rapidly.

In the beginning, you may not even be able to ski top to bottom and make continuous turns. If you can't, divide the mountain or run into manageable sections, increasing the distance until you can make it in one try.

Skiing in this manner will increase both the aerobic demands of the sport and your leg strength. You will not only maximize the benefits of skiing as an exercise, but your skiing will improve rapidly.

To maintain your fitness using skiing as your base activity, follow these guidelines:

*Day One*—Long, slow distance skiing at 65 to 70 percent of your maximal heart rate for at least forty-five continuous minutes
*Day Two*—Long, slow distance ski workout
*Day Three*—Long, slow distance ski or antigravity sport workout
*Day Four*—Long, slow distance ski workout
*Day Five*—Long, slow distance or modified speedplay skiing workout
*Day Six*—Long, slow distance ski or antigravity sport workout
*Day Seven*—Recreational skiing or rest

## The Training Program

Skiers interested in competition should have a very good aerobic base prior to the intensive three-month training program. The training program itself consists of four basic, long slow distance workouts and STEP and three interval and strength workouts.

The strength workout begins with twenty minutes of easy aerobics, either cycling or jogging. Follow it with the circuit resistive exercises in Chapter 9 and ten minutes of balancing exercises. Next, go to the stationary bicycle and do overloads by beginning at a low tension and pedaling for eighty to ninety revolutions per minute for sixty seconds. After a sixty-second rest period, increase the tension by one level. Continue this process until you can't maintain the eighty to ninety revolutions per minute for sixty seconds. This should happen after between five and eight work periods. Follow it with up to four minutes of wall-sits and five minutes of the penguin walk.

For intervals, run hills or stairs inside a gym or, if you can, outside. Refer to the interval chart, and find a hill that accommodates this kind of workout.

Start with twenty minutes of easy aerobics, and then about fifteen to twenty minutes of downhill eccentric exercise, either hopping down the stairs side to side or making S-turns down the hill. After half the workout, change the work period to the uphill segment and the rest period to downhill. As a variation, use hand weights or a weight vest for the intervals. The training schedule should be as follows:

*Day One*—Long, slow distance ski workout
*Day Two*—Interval workout
*Day Three*—Long, slow distance ski workout
*Day Four*—Strength workout
*Day Five*—Long, slow distance ski workout
*Day Six*—Interval workout
*Day Seven*—Long, slow distance ski workout

## The Cool-Down

Ski at an easy pace for five to ten minutes, and stretch as soon as you remove your skis.

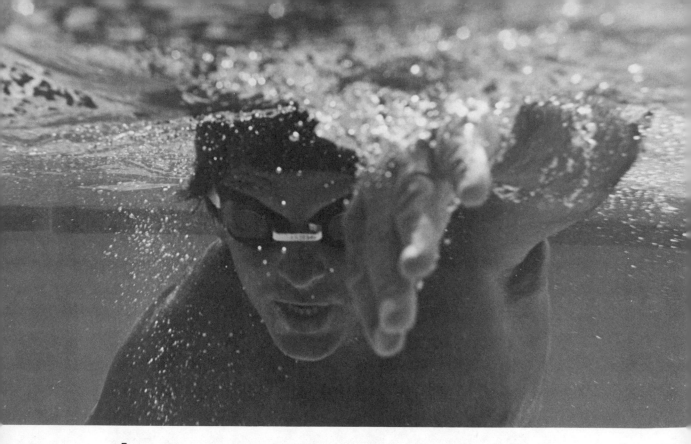

I T is always interesting for me to examine the way fitness myths develop. Despite much evidence to the contrary, for instance, jogging and running are widely believed to be so bad for the joints and skeletal system that many people shun the activities entirely. Swimming, on the other hand, has the reputation of being both safe (it is) and the best total body exercise (it isn't).

Perhaps swimming has had almost magical properties ascribed to it because immersing yourself in the water is invigorating and emotionally cleansing. After you get out of the pool or ocean, you feel refreshed and rejuvenated. This feeling is easily confused with the perception that you have had a good workout.

# 8 Swimming

This impression is further fostered by the widely repeated but inaccurate observation that swimming is the best possible aerobic activity. Despite its reputation as a total body sport, swimming is primarily an upper body sport. The legs provide some propulsion, but the muscle mass of the upper body is responsible for most of the motion. Since the key to aerobic activity is the extent of muscle mass used, swimming is obviously not as good an aerobic activity as, for example, cross-country skiing, which involves all the body's muscles to a much greater degree.

To a certain extent, swimming's antigravity nature also works against it. Depending on the individual's quantity of body fat (which is almost always greater in women than in men and thus makes this issue particularly important to female swimmers), water provides a considerable amount of buoyancy. This reduces the need to support the body in the water through muscle work, since relatively fatter people can lie in the water and float. Consequently, an hour in the pool can be like an hour's walk or an hour of golf—a pleasant experience, but not one that is aerobically demanding.

This is especially true for people who rely on a backyard pool for their workouts. These smaller pools are great for relaxation but not for exercise. For swimming to be aerobically effective, the pool should be at least twenty-five yards long. In anything shorter, you have to turn too much, and each turn becomes a little rest station. A mile in a fifty-meter Olympic pool is much more difficult, because it requires half as many turns, and thus provides half as much opportunity to rest.

Even if these turns were not a consideration, aerobic swimming in your backyard pool would be a gargantuan mental challenge. To complete a decent workout, you would have to swim hundreds of laps, making the exercise unbearably tedious and repetitive.

## Why Swim?

If you take these considerations into account, however, swimming can be a great activity. Among other things, it is perhaps the safest cornerstone to an effective aerobics program. As such, it is a welcome activity to those people already injured or worried about hurting themselves in their workouts.

About a year ago, for instance, a twenty-eight-year-old runner came to me with increasingly severe and debilitating knee pains. She had been competing in local 10k road races and doing very well in her age group. Then her knee pains forced her to stop running.

Her immediate problem was chondromalacia, or painful irritation of the inner surfaces of both patellae. The underlying cause of her problem, a condition known as malalignment syndrome, was even more troublesome. In this syndrome, which is more common in women due to their relatively wider hips, the kneecap is abnormally pulled sideways each time the quadriceps tighten. This causes the kneecap to grind against the thighbone, which often leads to chondromalacia and the accompanying knee pain.

Sometimes strengthening the quadriceps through specific exercises corrects this condition, and sometimes surgery is effective. At other times, as in this woman's case, malalignment syndrome is resistant to treatment and can be accommodated only by an exercise program that reduces the stresses around the knee joint.

As a dedicated runner, she was understandably despondent over having to give up running. After she made an unsuccessful attempt to substitute cycling, which also was painful for her, I suggested she begin swimming. She was skeptical but agreed to give it a chance. To her surprise, she enjoyed the sport, and was able to perform it without pain. Within a year, she was even ready to enter age-group competitions. By that time, she had been able to go back to very easy jogging but actually preferred swimming.

That's not to say that swimming is just for people who have been injured in their other endeavors. One of the country's best distance ocean swimmers stopped swimming during high school and started dancing, cycling, and running. As he approached his late twenties and found himself inundated with daily responsibilities, he returned to swimming. The solitude and tranquility of moving gracefully through the water for an hour a day was blissfully therapeutic. For him, as for many others, swimming provides an almost primal relaxation that no other exercise seems to bring.

An additional attraction is the challenge of learning how to swim properly. Although it usually is perceived as the simple act of putting one hand in front of the other, swimming, like running, involves a considerable degree of technical skill. Developing and refining this skill keeps many people from getting bored with what appears at first to be a repetitive sport.

Finally, once you have access to a pool or a body of water, swimming requires very little in the way of equipment. All that you really need are a pair of goggles so that you can open your eyes underwater without having them burn from the chlorine or salt, a tight-fitting nylon swimsuit that reduces the drag in the water, and, if necessary, a bathing cap that minimizes the drying effects chlorine can have on the hair.

## The Right Stroke

As in other sports, there is no substitute for formal swimming instruction. Advice on stroke frequency, breathing technique, kicking, and other matters of swimming form are best dealt with by swimming coaches. Here, however, are three tips which vastly improved my own performance and enjoyment of the sport.

The first involves how you place your hand in the water. Put your thumb in the water first, before your other fingers. This increases your power because it reduces the tendency to suppinate, or roll your hand outward so that it knifes through the water. Think of your hand as a paddle blade: when turned sideways, it slides through the water, but when turned correctly, it provides propulsion.

Next, just after your hand enters the water, imagine that there is a rope going underneath the center of your body from your head to your toes, which your hand must follow as it makes the stroke. The pulling motion that results

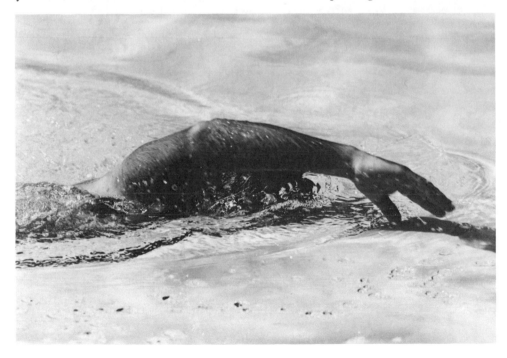

Entering the water, thumbs down

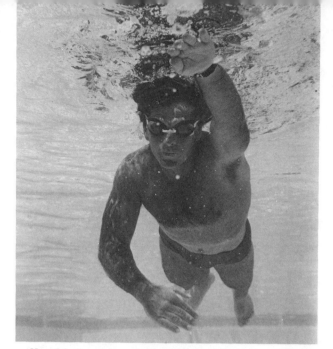

Pulling the rope

will add force to your efforts. Next, don't finish the stroke too early. Concentrate instead on pushing your extended arm past the lower abdomen. As the stroke finishes, your hand should brush by your thigh, taking advantage of the important propulsion at the end.

Obviously, there is more to swimming technique than these three hints. Nonetheless, making sure that you place your hand correctly, pull on the "rope," and push through the entire range of motion on the stroke should dramatically improve your swimming.

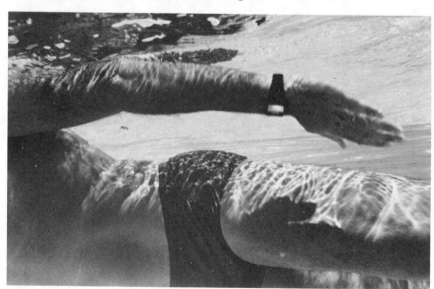

Pushing past the thigh

# Making Swimming Aerobic—and Interesting

Technique notwithstanding, the most important initial challenge with swimming is making your swimming workout fun and aerobic. This is especially important if, like most of us, you don't have access to Hawaiian lagoons or Caribbean beaches. More likely, your alternative will be that very boring rectangle we call a swimming pool.

A good solution is to join one of the excellent swimming classes offered by the YMCAs throughout the country, or those offered by colleges or the departments of parks and recreation. Like aerobics dance classes, they provide the stimulation, motivation, and support of a group. In addition, they teach you a variety of strokes, improve your performance, and effectively structure your workouts.

If you don't have the inclination to join such a class, there are still things you can do to make swimming more fun. Like the jogger who ambles mindlessly over the same course day in and day out, most swimmers dive into the water and swim the same number of laps the same way time after time. As we saw with running, the usual result of this pattern is burn out.

Swimming presents even more of a problem in this regard because you probably won't be able to regularly change the locale of your swimming program. Your only alternative is to vary the intensity and pattern of the workouts, as well as the strokes that you use.

To do that, divide the workout the same way you would any other, with a warm-up segment of ten minutes, an aerobic segment of thirty to sixty minutes, and a cool-down. Warm up by swimming at a relaxed pace for ten minutes. Swimming is so safe that you warm up less to prevent injury than to prevent early exhaustion. As with any other exercise, beginning the workout at an overly intense pace will require a great deal of anaerobic metabolism in the muscles that could lead to premature muscle fatigue.

Just as with the other aerobic activities, long slow distances make up the bulk of the workout program. Although you won't have any visual distractions during the workouts, you can make them more enjoyable by playing little games with yourself from day to day. One day, for instance, swim ten to twenty lengths freestyle at a moderate (65 to 70 percent of your maximal heart rate) pace. Then, after the tenth or twentieth lap, do the sidestroke, breaststroke, or elementary backstroke for the next two laps. Return to the crawl for the next ten or twenty laps, and then change the stroke for the following two laps, repeating the process until the sixty minutes are up.

At your next workout, do a modified speedplay workout. Make every tenth lap an all-out sprint, and follow it with two laps of breaststroke, sidestroke, or backstroke for recovery. Or after the warm-up, swim one to four lengths at a hard (but not exhausting) pace and recover for one length. Vary the subsequent lengths of the work period, recovering after each one for as long as is necessary. Make sure not to swim too hard and fatigue to the point that you can't complete the workout.

Serious swimmers have developed many other techniques to make the workouts more interesting. Of these, the best two are the broken swim and the ladder. In the broken swim, the number of laps is divided into segments that decrease by one lap. It takes sixty-six laps, for instance, to swim a swimmer's mile (fifteen hundred meters) in a twenty-five-yard pool. Break these laps into segments of eleven laps, ten laps, nine laps, eight laps, and on down to one lap. Swim each segment, stopping for ten to fifteen seconds in between each one, until the eleven segments are completed. Counting this way provides a psychological boost because the increasingly shorter segments are perceived as being easier than the preceding ones.

The ladder is another variation on the swimmer's mile. It divides the workouts into multiples of a certain number. A ladder of four laps, for example, is composed of segments of four, eight, twelve, and sixteen laps. To swim it, do four laps and rest for fifteen to thirty seconds. Next, swim eight laps and rest; then twelve and rest; and sixteen, and rest. Then go back down the ladder, swimming twelve laps and resting; eight laps and resting; and, finally, four laps and resting.

Although it may take beginning or slower swimmers about forty-five minutes to complete the broken swim or the ladder, more experienced or faster swimmers will do the fifteen hundred meters in under twenty minutes. If you can complete the distance in less than thirty to forty-five minutes, add segments of thirteen and twelve laps to the broken swim and twenty laps to the top of the ladder. Or use increments of two in the ladder, swimming two, four, six, eight, ten, and twelve laps and then ten, eight, six, four, and two. Adding extra segments extends the workout to its required length.

### Intervals

You can also do intervals in the pool. Like intervals in other sports, the ratio of the work to rest periods is critical. One- to three-minute work periods still apply, but to save yourself the difficulty of keeping time in the water, use the number of laps you can swim in that time as your standard. If you can swim four twenty-five-yard laps in sixty seconds, measure the interval in four laps, not sixty seconds. In that way, you won't have to worry about stopping in the middle of a lap.

Also, don't try to recover by swimming a lap, since an entire length may be too long for the recovery period. Try to finish the interval at the shallow end of the pool, where you can stand, keep time with a clock or your watch, and move around slowly as you prepare for the next interval.

## Swimming in STEP

For a long time, weight training was thought to be a good adjunct to competitive swimming. Traditions die as hard in athletics as they do anywhere else; even today, many competitive swimmers still lift weights. A recent study performed at the US Olympic Training Center, however, revealed that certain weight training exercises had a negative correlation with swimming ability. The better the swimmers were at reaching overhead and pulling down a weight, the worse they were at pulling themselves through the water with one swimming stroke. The better they were on the weights, in other words, the worse they were in the water.

It is no doubt possible to develop a weight-training program that improves your swimming performance, but this study demonstrates the importance of concentrating on exercises that are very specific to your sport. For swimming, one such exercise is the use of hand paddles. They come in different sizes, slip on the hand, and increase resistance through the water.

The paddles are also beneficial because they magnify the idiosyncracies and quirks of your stroke. If the stroke is not performed correctly, the paddles result in a jerky, uncomfortable motion. In addition to increasing the resistance, then, the paddles are great for improving your technique.

Swimming with the paddles is tiring, so save them for the last twenty to thirty minutes of the workout on days when you are concentrating on improving your strength. The first few times you use them, you will be able to swim only at a slow pace. But after working out with them for a while, you will be able to achieve a more intense pace.

Swimming with a pool buoy between your legs is another way to develop arm strength. The buoy prevents the legs from developing any propulsion and forces the arms to do all the work. Competitive swimmers make the exercise even harder by placing a small tire around their legs. The drag that results forces them to work still harder to get from one end of the pool to the other. The pool buoy exercises, which make swimming quite difficult, should be done at least once a week, either after you finish working with the paddles or during the last ten to fifteen minutes of the paddle-swim.

The drag suit, a bathing suit with pockets that was developed by Doc Councilman, is yet another way to increase the difficulty of a swimming workout. It traps water in its pockets, thus increasing the drag and the amount of effort required to propel you through the water. Although it is effective, it is less easily obtained than the paddles or the buoys.

To improve your kick and strengthen your upper thigh and hip muscles, hold a kickboard in your arms and propel yourself only by kicking. Alternate laps between the freestyle and frog kick. Don't waste your energy by splashing around; use your legs to smoothly kick through a full range of motion. Most people cannot maintain this exercise for more than ten to fifteen minutes. Ten minutes of legs-only swimming two to three times a week, however, can help make you a much stronger swimmer.

## The Workouts

To make sure that your workout is aerobically effective, monitor your heart rate throughout the exercise session. This is important for all but the most advanced swimmers, who through practice have learned to judge the intensity of their workouts. Less-experienced swimmers face the problem of sensory deprivation in the water, which is not present in dry-land sports. Performing the talk test while swimming, for example, is not recommended. Monitoring your heart rate is the only way to know if you are working out at the appropriate intensity. Even if you are an accomplished swimmer, monitor your heart rate during the first few weeks of training to make sure you're in the best range.

## The Maintenance Program

For a maintenance program that uses swimming as its base, follow these guidelines:

**Day One**—Broken swim at 65 to 70 percent of the maximal heart rate

**Day Two**—Jogging or cycling at 65 to 70 percent of the maximal heart rate, followed by optional circuit resistive exercises

**Day Three**—The ladder swim at 65 to 70 percent of the maximal heart rate

**Day Four**—Jogging or cycling at 65 to 70 percent of the maximal heart rate, followed by optional circuit resistive exercises

**Day Five**—One-hour swim at 65 to 70 percent of the maximal heart rate, making every tenth lap a full-out sprint, followed by one lap of side, breast, or elementary backstroke for recovery

**Day Six**—A skill sport workout, such as tennis or aerobic dance, or long, slow jogging or cycling with optional circuit resistive exercises

**Day Seven**—An extended ladder swim plus STEP

If you insist on using swimming as the only activity in your training program, replace day two with twenty to thirty minutes of easy swimming and an interval workout, day four with a broken swim, and day five with twenty to thirty minutes of easy swimming and a second interval workout.

## The Training Program

Competitive swimming is well organized in the United States, so there are numerous races in the half-mile to mile category that you can participate in. To find out when and where the races are held, ask your local university, junior college, or Y for the local Swim Masters' organization. They sponsor the various races, and also give you the chance to swim with people of your own age and ability.

Training for these races is much like training for a 5K or a 10K in running. In the first two weeks of the three-month period it takes to peak, do speedplay workouts without worrying about the ratio of work to rest times. Swim for two or six laps at 85 to 90 percent of your maximal heart rate, and take as long as necessary to recover, swimming hard again only when you are ready.

During these two weeks, alternate three speedplay workouts per week with long, slow distance workouts. To get the benefits of cross training, however, consider interspersing them with two jogging or cycling workouts and one STEP workout.

## Weeks one and two

For weeks one and two, a good training schedule would be:

**Day One**—Broken swim
**Day Two**—Speedplay swimming workout
**Day Three**—Ladder swim or long, slow distance cycling or jogging
**Day Four**—Speedplay swimming workout
**Day Five**—Broken swim or long, slow distance cycling or jogging workout
**Day Six**—Speedplay swimming workout
**Day Seven**—One-hour swim, followed by STEP workout

## Weeks three through ten

In these weeks you will make use of interval training, so don't forget the basic principle of intervals, which is that the work period must be at least twice as long as the rest period.

Interval workouts are, or should be, very intense, so do them only twice a week. Never do an interval workout unless you are properly rested. A good guideline is to give yourself a minimum of two days between interval training sessions. So that you don't burn out, don't push yourself too hard too fast. Begin by picking intensities in the easiest ranges, and work up to the more difficult ones in the sixth or seventh week.

Alternate the intervals with two long, slow distance swimming workouts and two long, slow distance cycling or running workouts. On the seventh day, do repeats, which will help you peak and refine your racing technique. To do them, swim from one to four laps at close to maximum pace, then swim slowly and begin the process again only when you are fully recovered. Over the training period, increase the number of laps until by its end you can swim four-lap segments for the entire workout. During this period, your workout schedule should look like this:

**Day One**—Broken swim

*Day Two*—Thirty minutes of easy swimming, followed by intervals

*Day Three*—Long, slow distance cycling or jogging, followed by optional circuit resistive exercises

*Day Four*—Ladder swim

*Day Five*—Thirty minutes of easy swimming, followed by intervals

*Day Six*—Long, slow distance cycling or jogging, followed by optional circuit resistive exercises

*Day Seven*—Twenty to thirty minutes of easy swimming, followed by twenty to thirty minutes of repeats

## Weeks eleven and twelve

In this tapering phase, you are no longer concerned with building cardiopulmonary power. Instead, use modified repeats to sharpen your form and technique. Swim at a race pace for one to four laps; recover for one to four laps; swim at race pace for one to four laps; recover for one to four laps; until the workout is over. Visualize yourself actually in the race side by side with other swimmers during the work periods. This will help prepare you psychologically and physiologically for the event.

In the eleventh week, do one interval and two repeat workouts, alternating them with long, slow distances. Use this schedule as a guideline:

*Day One*—Broken swim

*Day Two*—Repeats

*Day Three*—Long, slow distance running or cycling workout

*Day Four*—Thirty-minute swim, followed by intervals

*Day Five*—Ladder swim

*Day Six*—Repeats

*Day Seven*—Long, slow distance running or cycling workout

If you are carbo-loading during the twelfth week (see Appendix 5), use the following workout schedule for the last week of training:

*Day One*—A two-hour swim at a moderately high intensity

*Day Two*—Thirty-minute easy swim, run, or cycling workout

*Day Three*—Thirty-minute easy swim workout

*Day Four*—Thirty-minute easy ladder

*Day Five*—Thirty-minute easy broken swim

***Day Six***—Thirty-minute easy repeats
***Day Seven*** (Prerace)—Rest

If you are not carbo-loading or are training for an event that is not a marathon or ultra-endurance (over two hour) event, alternate two repeats with two long, slow distance swimming workouts and two long, slow distance running or cycling workouts as follows:

***Day One***—Broken swim
***Day Two***—Long, slow distance cycling or running workout
***Day Three***—Repeats
***Day Four***—Ladder swim
***Day Five***—Long, slow distance running or cycling workout
***Day Six***—Repeats
***Day Seven***—Fifteen to twenty minutes easy swimming

## The Cool-Down

After the aerobic segment of the workout, spend about five minutes swimming at a slow, relaxed pace. Swimming is much more of a loosening than a tightening activity compared to other sports. Even so, swimmers can benefit from a good stretching program that is regularly performed after this cool-down phase.

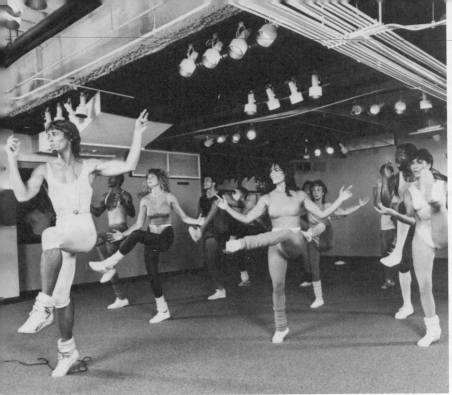
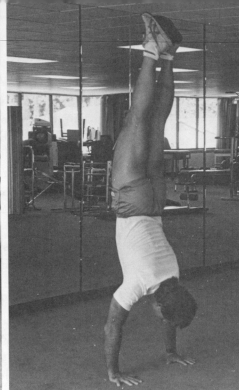

ONE of the most popular and enjoyable exercise activities of the last five years is the "aerobics" class. Popularized by people like Jane Fonda and Richard Simmons, the "dance" appellation frequently coupled with the word "aerobics" is due to the dance-type movements incorporated in these classes. Whether by design or accident, the use of choreographed dance steps seems to have been a very clever idea, because it immediately added elegance to an activity which might otherwise have been nothing more than jumping about in an enclosed room.

Learning how to move gracefully is only one of the many assets of these classes. A second key ingredient is their group nature. The psychological support provides a powerful stimulus to emulate, not unlike the effect one

# Aerobic Dancing and Resistive Exercise 9

person can have clapping in an audience. Best of all, you actually have someone at the front of the room showing you what to do. Add to these reasons convenience and pulsing music, and it is not hard to understand why aerobics is the national pastime for an estimated twenty million Americans and is still growing.

Yet as with any emerging activity, there are a number of problems that should be addressed. The first of these, ironically, is making sure that the classes are truly aerobic. One of the most successful "aerobic" videotapes, in fact, had less than two minutes of aerobic activity. Remember the three basic ingredients of aerobic exercise: most of the body's muscle mass must be working; the heart must beat at least 65 percent of its maximum; and the exercise must be sustained for at least fifteen minutes. Most people are in aerobics classes to lose weight, and thus require sustained aerobic activity of thirty to sixty minutes, so this is a serious concern.

Another problem area is the toning exercises, which often comprise half or more of the class. They are often taken to be synonymous with spot reduction, or selectively removing fat from unwanted places by exercising adjacent muscles. One of the most popular of these involves lying on the floor on the side and doing endless leg raises. While this will tone and strengthen the muscles responsible for accomplishing the motion, it won't remove fat from the hips. The only way to diminish the quantity of fat in our bodies is by stimulating the body's metabolism, not by vibrating, pounding, or fatiguing adjacent muscles.

If you are not convinced of this, just take a look at marathon runners. From an aesthetic point of view, they may not have the most attractive physiques, but they are certainly the leanest of any group of people. And they become lean not by exercising one muscle to fatigue but by working all their muscles simultaneously over long periods of time. They clearly demonstrate that the way to a lean body is through total body exercise.

Although the classes are effective at toning muscles, they are not as effective as they could be. The failure in large part comes from a reliance on exercises that cause you to move only through a small range of motion and, as a result, call into play only a small number of motor units in the muscles involved.

To understand why this is a shortcoming, think back on the stories you may have heard concerning people who were able to lift cars that their children were trapped under or do other seemingly incredible feats of strength.

These stories, many of which are documented, demonstrate that our musculoskeletal system has strength potential that is truly astounding.

Although all of us have a huge potential reserve, we use only a tiny fraction of our muscle motor units most of the time. One of the goals of strength exercise, or exercise that increases muscle girth, is the stimulation of as many of the motor units available to us as possible. We may never reach the muscle recruitment levels possible during moments of acute terror, but we can certainly stimulate more muscle mass than the exercises in the classes do.

You are probably wondering either why the classes would rely on this limited range of motion exercises or why, if they are not effective, the exercises seem so hard. Strangely enough, the answer to both questions is the same. Because the exercises utilize only a small number of motor units in the muscle, they fatigue very quickly. As they do, you get the mildly painful sensation, or "burn," that is held in such reverence by misinformed teachers.

This fatigue, or burn, however, is ultimately a fake fatigue. You haven't used, much less exhausted, enough muscle mass to matter, nor have you developed anything approaching maximal tension in it. As a result, you may very well feel like you have had a workout, but your actual strength gains will be minimal.

## Improving on the Class

To make your workout more effective, you have to be willing to be a little different from the rest of the class, even if that means being embarrassed, or "corrected" by the teacher, who has a vested interest in having the class stick to his routines. The first way you will improve on the class is by substituting large motions for the smaller movements favored by the teachers.

When the teacher tells the class to do small circles with the arms, for instance, make full ones. Since circling the arms in a big motion uses greater muscle mass than the small circles, it will make the exercise more aerobically effective. Also, during these exercises, many teachers tell their class to keep the wrists taut so that the hand points either down or up, with the forearm muscles shortened. When short, however, muscles have very little ability to develop tension, so this rationale is misguided in that it does not

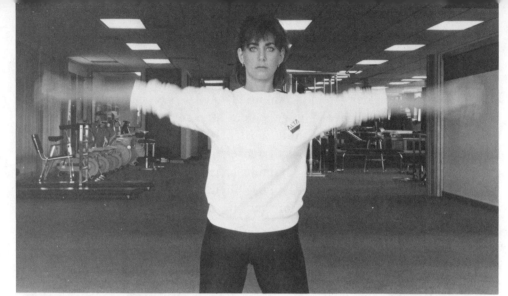

Small,
ineffective arm
circles

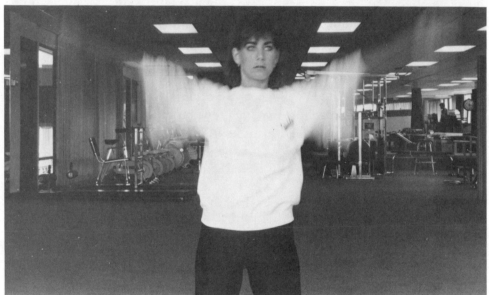

Big, effective
arm circles

add to strength gains. Pointing your hand up or down may have some appeal of form to a purist, but no practical function.

Similarly, exercises that concentrate on the abdominal region are very important to an exercise program. Many aerobics classes advocate small ranges of motion, the so-called abdominal crunches, but they are not as effective as the more traditional sit-ups detailed later in this chapter. The most powerful muscles for flexing the trunk (moving your chest to your knees) are the muscles that attach between the spine and the thighbone (femur).

The muscle that runs from the front of the ribs to the pelvic bone (the rectus abdominus) is actually an accessory muscle of trunk flexion. Exercises which concentrate on only the rectus abdominus, such as the crunches, omit the most important muscles of trunk flexion.

Hard evidence in support of this was recently published by Swedish physiologist Alf Thorstensen in a study of Swedish Air Force recruits both with and without low back pain. The group with low back pain had much weaker hip, or lower trunk, flexors than the normal group. Since the more traditional sit-ups work these muscles as well as the rectus abdominus, they are more effective both at rehabilitating as well as preventing low back pain.

Keeping as many muscles as possible working, even when the rest of the class is concentrating on only one muscle, is another way to improve the class. For example, when the running segment ends and the teacher begins the arm exercises, keep your feet moving in time to the music and the arm movements. Remember the golden rule of aerobics: the more muscles that are working simultaneously, the more aerobic the exercise becomes.

Still another way to make the class more effective is by coming into it already warm. Despite the recently discovered dangers of pre-activity stretching, most aerobics teachers still insist on beginning their classes with a stretching segment. If you come into the class without having warmed up first, you risk minor muscle strains. By getting on a stationary bicycle or shuffle-jogging around the block for ten minutes before class, you can come in already warmed up and thus eliminate any of these dangers.

By doing so, you will also get a head start on the aerobics segment of the class. If the aerobic content of the class doesn't keep you within the target heart rate of 65 to 70 percent of your maximal heart rate for at least thirty minutes, you should spend additional time jogging, swimming, or cycling either on a stationary bike or on the road so that you can get a workout that is fat-burning.

## Preventing Injuries

Some studies suggest that at least 65 percent of the people who take aerobics classes have or have had at least one injury that can be traced directly to the class itself. This is not surprising considering that the exercises involved are heavily eccentric, and are often done on poorly designed floors.

There is very little you can do to eliminate the eccentric motion of the class, primarily because you move around in a very small amount of space. This restricted area makes aerobic dancing much more eccentric than running, in which you can reduce the amount of eccentric activity by eliminating up-and-down motion and incorporating heel-to-toe movements into your stride. Ideally, aerobics teachers would not rely on jumping jacks or running in place, but use the entire room for the running segment of the class.

The most common problems occurring in the classes are Achilles tendinitis, shin splints (generalized pain along the shin bone), ankle sprains, plantar fasciitis, and occasionally stress fractures. One of the best preventive measures you can take is to wear an aerobic shoe with good absorption qualities and good side-to-side support.

Although that almost seems like unnecessary advice, many people still go into a class without giving much thought, if any, to what type of shoe they should wear. A nationally known aerobics instructor, for instance, came to me with pain under the balls of her feet. After examining her, I saw that the problem was in the metatarsal arch of the balls of her feet. At the time, she did not wear shoes during the aerobics classes, apparently because she liked the freedom and feeling of grace and elegance that going barefoot brought. After a period of rest in which the injury healed, she became very careful about wearing the proper footgear and resumed her classes without any additional problems.

Don't make the mistake of thinking that you can get away with a pair of leg warmers, either, because they are not useful for anything other than the dance look. By themselves they cannot prevent shin splints or any of the other lower leg problems. As fashionable as they may be, they don't provide enough warmth to protect the muscles. They can help retain heat once it is generated, but they won't supply heat by themselves. Besides, shin splints are not caused by cold muscles but by the repetitive, eccentric nature of the aerobics classes. Warming up is important but cannot prevent problems caused by the nature of the class.

Injuries also occur because of fatigue. In fact, one of the most popular hip exercises regularly sends people to my sports medicine clinic. These hip exercises isolate the muscles that are responsible for abducting the leg, or lifting it sideways. The misguided reason for this exercise, of course, is spot reduction of the cottage cheese dimples that are caused by the fat deposits around the hips. Remind yourself that it is total body exercise, not isolated hip motions, that will remove this fat.

Isolating the hip muscles and fatiguing them in this heavily eccentric exercise not only does not work but also, at a certain point, makes the muscle susceptible to injury. Unfortunately, that point varies from individual to individual and cannot be predicted in advance. A simple way to avoid the problem is by doing hip circles, moving the straight leg in a circle as it is raised, as opposed to moving up and down.

Even if you followed all this advice, it still would be difficult to develop an effective training program using aerobic dancing as your only aerobic activity. That is not to say that it cannot be done; just that it generally isn't. Instead of concentrating solely on the classes, use the fun of the group, the music, and the pleasant surroundings of the classes to motivate you to exercise. But don't make the mistake of concentrating too much on them. Take three or four classes a week and supplement them with other activities, such as swimming, cycling, easy jogging, or cross-country skiing. If, like many of the people in the classes, you are interested in improving your appearance, do the circuit resistive exercises that follow twice a week. They will help build lean body mass in the form of more developed muscles.

As of yet, there is very little organized competition and practically no mass aerobics competition, so competitive training goals and peaking are terms that don't really apply here. To maintain fitness, however, schedule your workouts as follows:

## The Workouts

*Day One*—Ten minutes of shuffle-jogging or cycling, followed by the class. Take your heart rate frequently; if you are not working at 65 to 70 percent of your maximal heart rate for at least thirty minutes, follow the class with a long, slow distance running, cycling, or swimming workout.

*Day Two*—Long, slow distance in any aerobic activity besides an aerobics class and circuit resistive exercises

*Day Three*—Ten minutes of shuffle-jogging or cycling, followed by the class and, if necessary, a long, slow distance workout at an aerobic activity of your choice

*Day Four*—Long, slow distance in any aerobic activity besides an aerobics class and circuit resistive exercise

**Day Five**—Ten minutes of shuffle-jogging or cycling, followed by the class and, if necessary, a long, slow distance workout at an aerobic activity of your choice

**Day Six**—Long, slow distance in any aerobic activity besides a class and, if necessary, a long, slow distance workout at an aerobic activity of your choice

**Day Seven**—Rest or ten minutes of shuffle-jogging, swimming, or cycling, followed by the class and, if necessary, a long, slow distance workout at an aerobic activity of your choice

## The Resistive Exercise Circuit

Although many people have turned to expensive weight-training systems or free-weight workouts to build strength and muscle bulk, gymnasts, who use only their own bodies, prove conclusively that using your own body weight as the resistance can result in very strong and beautifully proportioned bodies. Another thing about using your own body as resistance is that very little apparatus is required. A few of the exercises, however, are more beneficial if you have access to a few pieces of equipment.

*The resistive exercise circuit that follows was designed for people who do not have access to a health club*. If you do, you can substitute analogous equipment stations for the following exercises. The bench press, for example, is an exercise analogous to push-ups. But you can get a complete workout by using these exercises, which require only your own body and several pieces of readily available apparatus.

Each of the following exercises should be done with a continuous rhythm and, unless otherwise stated, to comfortable fatigue. Specifically, if you can do less than twenty repetitions, the exercise is too difficult and should be made easier, as described below. Similarly, if you can do more than thirty, the exercise is too easy and should be made harder, as described below. The exercises are most effective when done in the order they are presented, as they are designed to work all the muscles of the body systematically and in complementary fashion. This is important because you can only develop body equilibrium by exercising muscles which oppose each other. If, for example, you do an exercise that develops your chest, it should be complemented by an exercise which develops your upper back.

Station One—Push-Ups. In the classical push-up, your arms will support

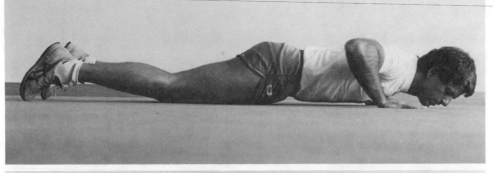

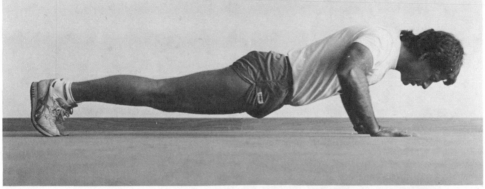

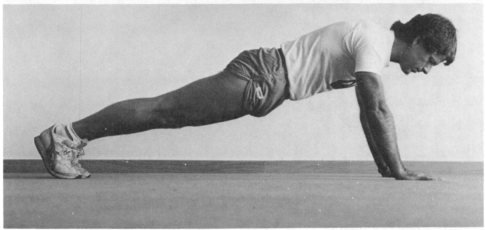

Regular push-ups

about 75 percent of your body weight. This may be too difficult for many people, especially women. To make the exercise easier, perform the push-ups standing up against a wall. Face the wall and place your hands in push-up position on it. Take one giant step backward, and do the push-ups from this position. Touch your chest to the wall with each push-up. These push-ups require much less strength than the classical push-ups.

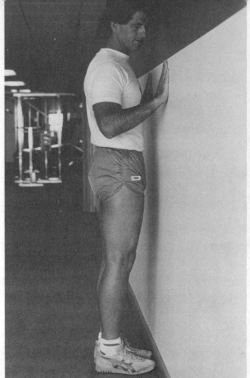

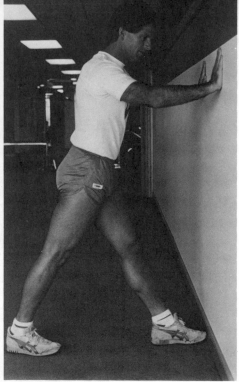

Easy wall
push-ups

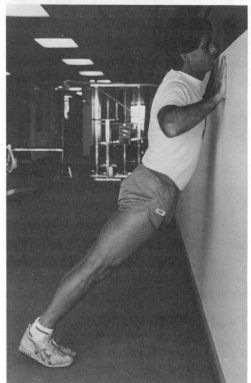

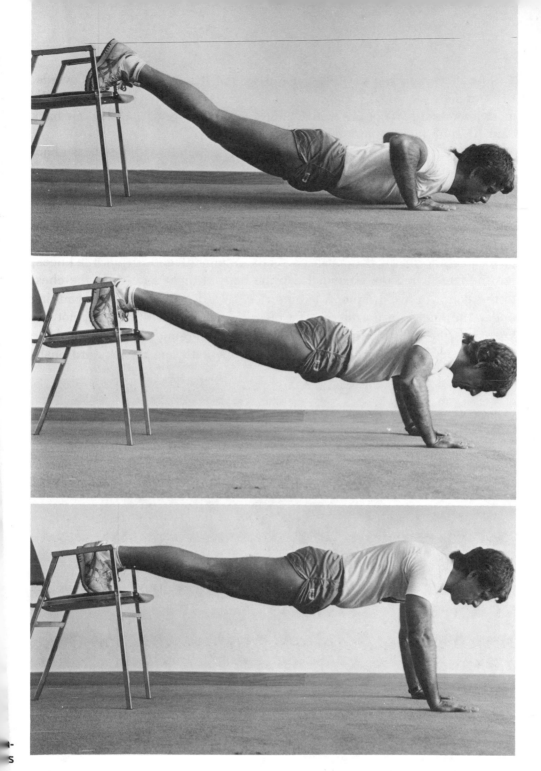

Note that when you do these push-ups, your back will arch back
Back arches, technically known as back extension exercises, are one
most important parts of preventive and rehabilitation programs for lo
pain, despite their reputation as being dangerous.

When or if these become very easy, use an armchair with armrest
shoulder width apart. Typically these armrests will be about two-and
feet above the ground. Place your hands on the armrests and do pu
between them. This forces you to lift slightly more of the body weig
the standing-up push-up, but less than floor push-ups.

When these become too easy, do the intermediate, or so-called
push-up or the classic floor push-up. In the intermediate push-up, th
not the feet, touch the ground. Keep the body straight and lower t
to the floor. To avoid minor knee injuries, wear knee pads or use
under the knees during these. The classic push-up uses the feet
knees, as the fulcrum, or point that touches the ground. When e
no longer challenge you, put your feet up on a chair and do stand

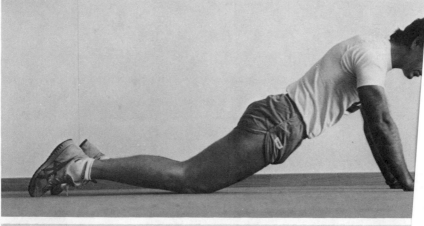

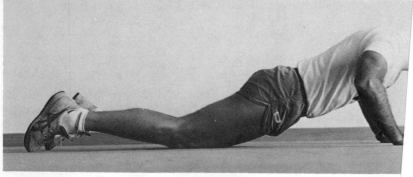

Difficult pus
u

ups from this position. This demands that you lift at least 85 percent of your body weight and thus is considerably more difficult than the floor push-ups.

Station Two—The Rowing Machine. If you don't have access to a rowing machine, you might consider buying one because it is a worthwhile and relatively inexpensive purchase. The two essential requirements for the machine are that it have a seat that moves freely back and forth with very little friction and that it have foot straps that hold your feet securely in place. Most of the models that are available provide resistance through some sort of hydraulic apparatus, usually cylindrical in shape, that is easily varied. This exercise is an excellent complement to the push-ups, and primarily develops the upper back muscles and, to a considerable extent, the arms. Unfortunately, the rowing machine is necessary for this station. If you don't have access to one, go directly from the push-ups to the abdominal exercises in the next station.

Station Three—Abdominal Exercises. The best abdominal exercises require an abdominal slant board with a means of securing the feet and ankles and of raising the height of the board to increase the exercise's resistance. If you don't have one, you can secure the feet underneath a couch, chair, or bed. When doing these, slightly bend the knees (but not so much that they are completely flexed). Start by sitting up. Lean backward until the torso almost touches the floor (or board). Then return to the up position.

Keep in mind that, as in all resistive exercises, the down motion is more eccentric and therefore potentially more dangerous. Thus, do the downward motion more slowly than the upward motion, especially at the beginning of the program.

The position of the hands and arms can be used to increase the resistance and difficulty of the exercise. The easiest position occurs when the slant board is horizontal and the hands are folded on the lower abdomen. To make the sit-ups slightly harder, fold the hands across the chest. Then, when these become too easy, place the hands behind the head.

The resistance can also be made more difficult by raising the level of the slantboard. In the absence of a board, increase the resistance by holding books or a weighted object either on the chest or placing them behind the head.

Notwithstanding what you may have learned elsewhere, it is very important to use a full range of motion in this exercise. Limiting the range does not develop a specific part of a muscle. It does, however, reduce the effectiveness

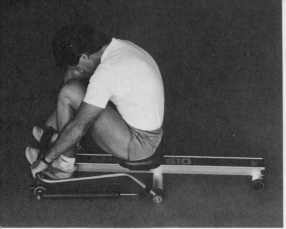

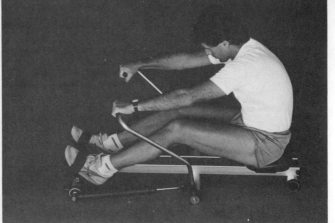

Rowing: The
starting
position
(*above left*)

The leg thrust
(*above right*)

The
back extension
(*center right*)

The arm pull
(*bottom right*)

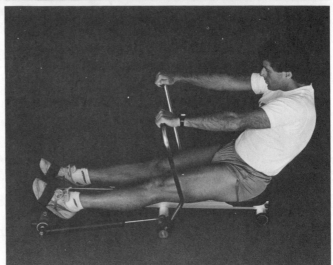

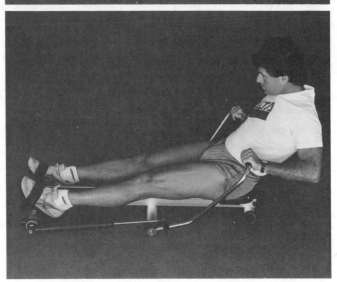

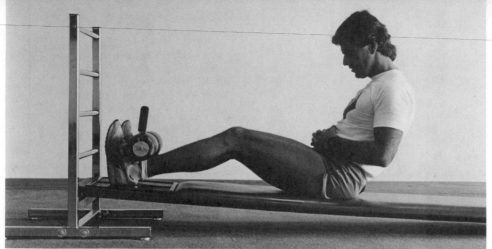

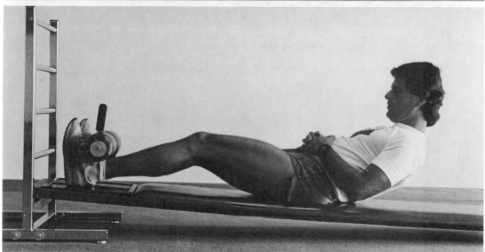

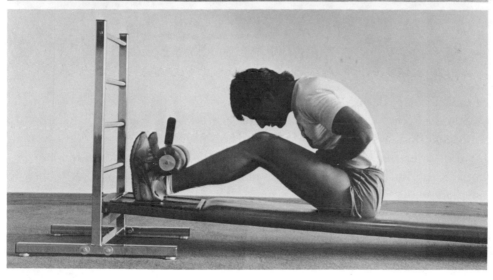

Easy sitbacks

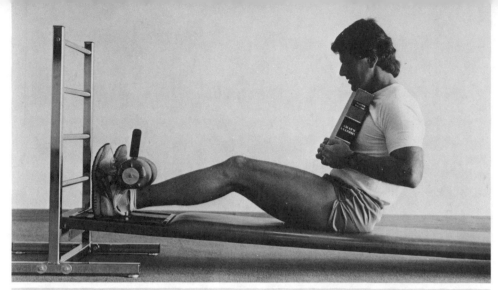

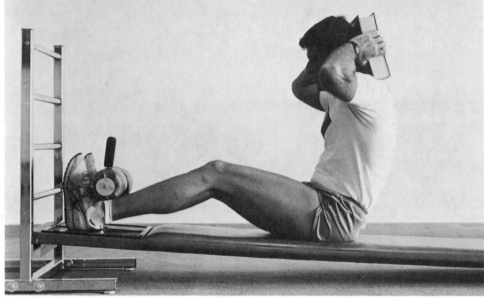

of the exercise, because it limits the recruitment of the muscles' motor units.

Station Four—Back Extension. Back exercises, or back arches, are very important but frequently overlooked. They provide much needed strength for the lower back and are an excellent complement to the abdominal exercises. If you have a slant board, raise it so that it is about six inches to no more than one foot off the ground. Then place a pad, such as a sofa cushion or pillow, on the slant board to support your thighs. Lie on the board face down, securing your feet in the strap or post that held your ankles. Do

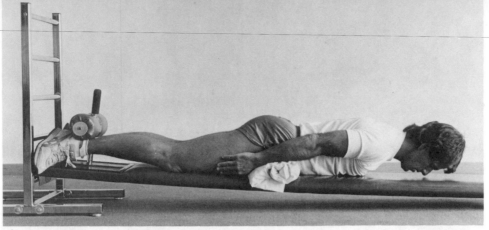

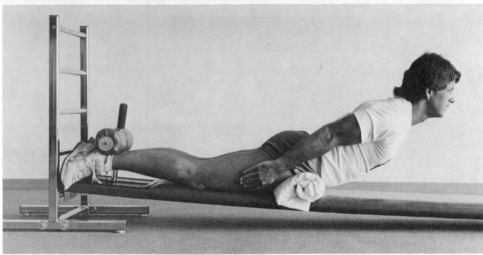

Back extension exercises with the slant board

back extensions by lifting the torso as far off the slant board as possible. The easiest way to do the exercise is by raising the slant board six inches off the ground. To make it harder, raise the board, place the hands behind the head, or hold books or a weighted object behind the head as you do the back extension.

If you don't have a slant board, take one or two sofa cushions and place them on the floor so that the upper thighs are supported up to the level of the hipbones. Lie on the floor face down, hook your feet under a sofa or bed, and do the back extensions from this position.

Station Five—Squat Thrusts. In a standing position, bend the legs and hang your arms straight down so that your fingertips touch the floor. Forcefully extend your body upward, straightening the knees and going up on your toes in one continuous movement. This exercise can be made more difficult by

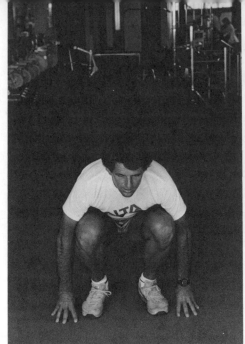

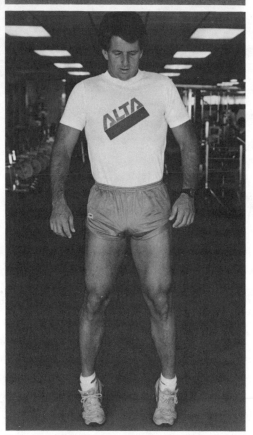

Squat thrusts

making the movement an actual jump or by holding a weighted object, such as dumbells or books, in the hands. If you hold an object, make sure it touches the floor with each repetition.

Station Six—The Military Press. To do this, you must have a strong table or chair that is secured against a wall or else so heavy that it is unlikely to move. If you have one, a standard-size table is ideal. Take one giant step away from it, and put your hands on its edge in standard push-up position. As your arms bend, let your head sink below the table's edge, touching the back of your neck to it. Then push away, in an action that is similar to a push-up.

To make the exercise more difficult, use a lower table (of equally sturdy dimensions). Then, when you get more advanced, raise your feet by supporting them on a chair or stool and do the exercise from this position. If you are exceptionally strong, you can even place your hands on the floor at approximately the distance from your elbow to your fingertips away from the wall, and do a handstand against the wall. Then do the military press from the handstand position.

Station Seven—Jump Rope. Skipping can be aerobic, but here it is used to develop the lower leg, primarily the calf, muscles. Jump for three minutes. Make the exercise harder by using a heavier rope or one with weighted handles. You can weight the handles yourself by wrapping the end of the handles with lead tape. Increasing the cadence and intensity of the skipping is another way of making the exercise more difficult.

Station Eight—Bar Dips. Usually performed between parallel bars a shoulder-width apart, the exercise can be made simpler by using a bench or strong chair as the apparatus. Place your hands on the bench behind your back, support your torso by placing your legs straight out on the floor in front of you, and bend your arms. As you do, your seat should sink as far to the floor as possible. Then come back up.

It may be more fun to work out with shiny, high-tech machines, but using your own body weight and these resistive exercises will develop strength in all major muscle groups of the body and will result in a well-proportioned physique. Again, when doing these exercises, do not rest between stations or repetitions. To be most effective, the motion should be continuous. When combined with an aerobic program that burns fat, they can be very effective in developing body strength and increasing lean body mass. Unlike aerobic activity, which should be done every day, these exercises will have their

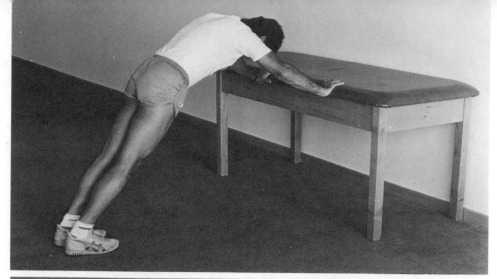

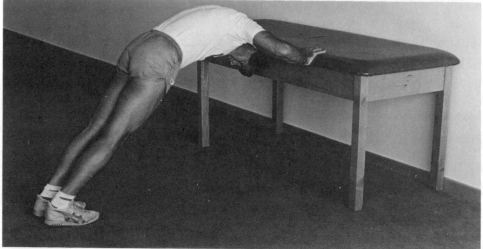

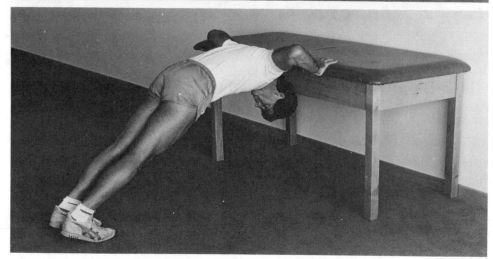

The basic
military press

maximum effectiveness if done vigorously three times a week, giving your body a chance to relax in between the sessions.

## Flexibility

From the discussion of stretching in Chapter 2, you already know how and when to stretch. If you don't have time to do each stretch below, perform those that affect the areas in which you have just exercised, where you traditionally hold tension (especially the muscles of the neck and shoulders), or where you feel tight. Make sure that you choose at least one stretch from each of the muscle groups, and that you vary the selection from day to day so that you don't avoid the stretch or stretches that are the hardest (and thus the most critical) for you.

Stretch only when you are warmed up and, preferably, only at the end of your workout. Remember to breathe in a relaxed manner during each stretch, gently extending the stretch as you exhale. Hold each stretch for at least a minute, and never do a stretch that is painful. While you want to produce some tension in the stretch, that tension should be low enough so that you can maintain it for the minute without pain. A stretch that is too intense will stimulate contraction, not relaxation, of the muscle and thus will not make you more flexible. Worse, overly intense stretching may result in minor muscle tears.

### The upper body stretches

1. The Neck Stretch—Sit in a chair and slowly drop your head so that your chin touches the chest. Clasp the hands behind the neck and allow the weight of the arms to slowly pull the head forward. Hold for a minute. Then tilt the head all the way back and let it hang for sixty seconds. Then slowly tilt the head to each side, holding each position for sixty seconds.

2. Sidebends—Stand with your feet a few inches apart. Lift your right arm over your head so that your right hand falls down behind your left shoulder. Grasp the right elbow with your left hand and tilt your body as far as you can to the left side. Hold for sixty seconds and then repeat on the opposite side.

3. Prayer Pose—Kneel. Sit back on your heels and bend at your hips so that your chest touches your knees. Stretch your arms out in front of you,

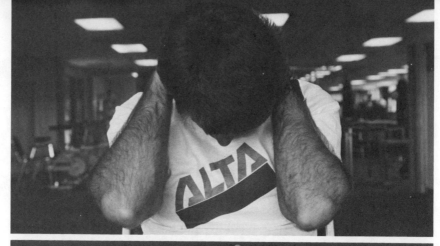

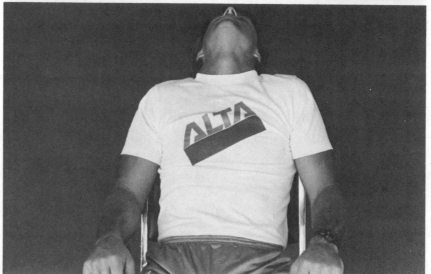

The neck
stretch

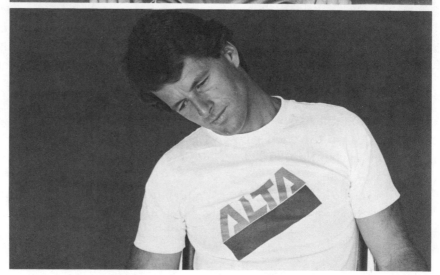

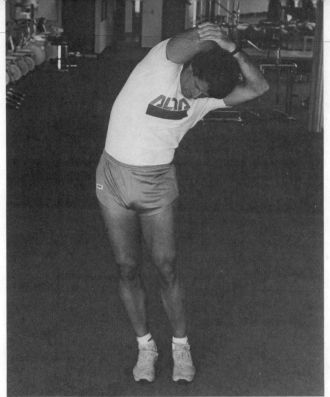

The side bend

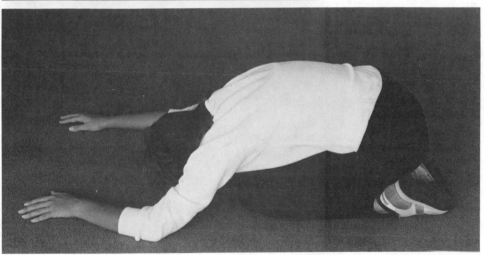

The prayer pose

relaxing your neck and resting your head on the floor. Stretch your arms out as far as you can.

4. Back Arch Stretch—Lie on your stomach with your hands beneath the shoulders. Extend the arms as if you were going to do a push-up, but allow the torso and the abdomen to sag on the floor. Arch the head and neck

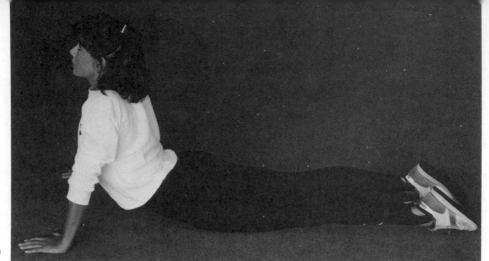

The back arch

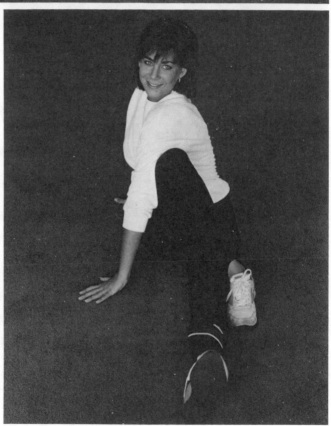

The rotator

backwards. Hold for sixty seconds. This stretch is particularly important for those with low back problems.

5. Rotator Stretches—Sit with your legs outstretched. Put the right foot

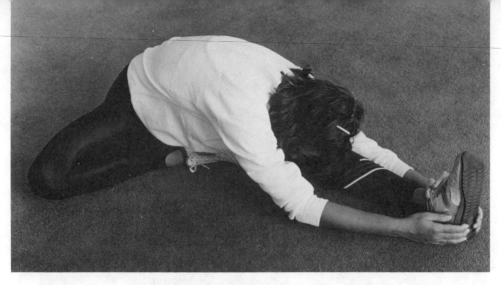

The hurdler

on the outside of the left knee. Place both hands on the right side of your body, twisting the torso so that you look over your right shoulder. Repeat on the opposite side.

### The hamstrings and lower back

1. Hurdler Stretches—Sit with one leg straight, toes pointed. Bend the other so that the sole of your foot touches the inside thigh of the straight leg. Take a deep breath, stretch your arms forward, and bend from the hip, reaching forward toward your toes as you exhale. Relax your torso as much as possible, so that it sags forward and down onto the outstretched leg. Hold for sixty seconds, and then slowly unwind. Return to the sitting position and repeat with the opposite leg.

2. Butterfly Stretch—Sit with your knees bent and the soles of your feet touching each other. Allow the knees to fall to the outside as you grasp your feet and attempt to bring your torso between your thighs. Gently press the legs toward the floor as you simultaneously let your torso sag between your thighs. Hold for sixty seconds.

### The ankle and calf

1. The Achilles Stretch—Stand against a wall. Take one giant step backward with one foot. Leave the other foot against the wall. Keep the knee of your back leg straight and bend the front knee so that your hips move forward toward the wall. Hold for sixty seconds and then change feet.

2. Soleus Stretch—Squat with your feet together and your toes facing slightly out. Drop your head and torso onto your knees. Rock slightly forward

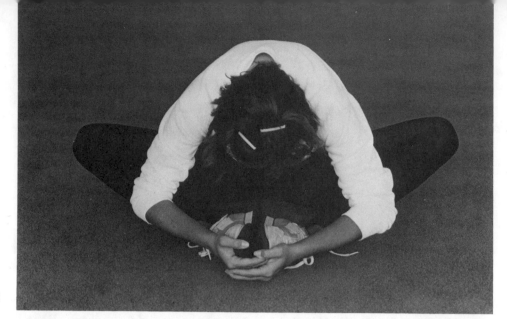

The butterfly

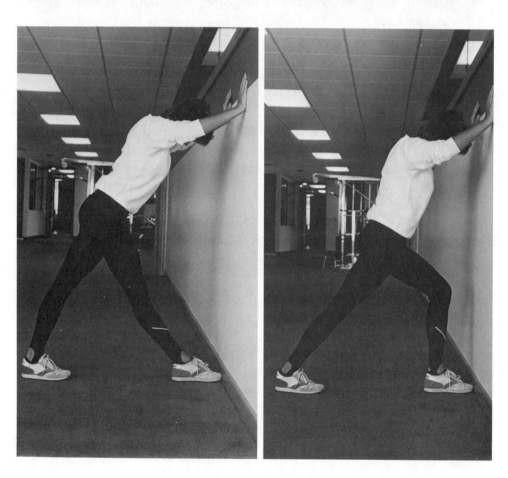

The Achilles stretch, with the back leg straight

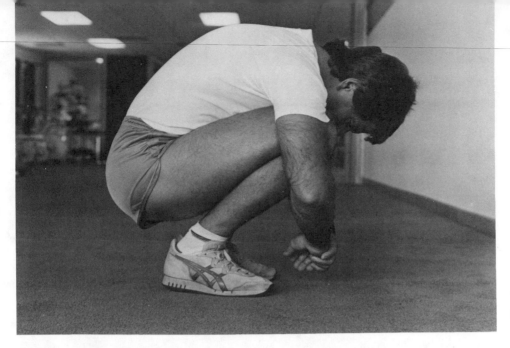

The soleus
stretch

onto the balls of the feet to increase tension to the appropriate level and hold for sixty seconds.

### All major muscle groups

1. The Sit and Reach—Sit on the floor with your legs outstretched and together. Place your hands behind the knees, calves, ankles, or feet, de-

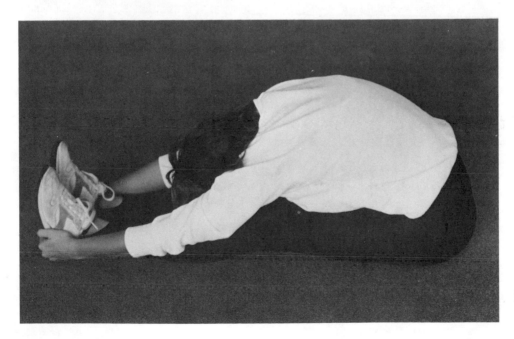

Sit and reach

pending on your degree of flexibility, and allow the torso to sag forward. Hold for sixty seconds.

Do the back arches and the sit and reach stretches every day. The side-bend, rotator, and Achilles stretch are particularly good for anyone involved in running or dance activities. These few simple stretches, done for five to ten minutes a day, will provide you will all the flexibility that you need. The other stretches are optional, and can be added to your program if you lack flexibility in those areas.

## Appendix 1—Maximum Predicted Heart Rate in Women and Men

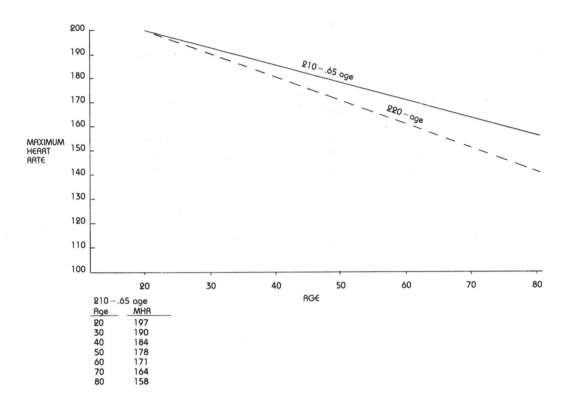

MAXIMUM HEART RATE

AGE

210 − .65 age

| Age | MHR |
|-----|-----|
| 20 | 197 |
| 30 | 190 |
| 40 | 184 |
| 50 | 178 |
| 60 | 171 |
| 70 | 164 |
| 80 | 158 |

The solid line is based on the formula $210 - .65$ of your age. Note the difference between it and the more commonly used but less-accurate formula $220 - $ your age, which is represented by the dotted line.

NOTE: Many people ask me why their heart rates are higher than the chart. All values, I explain, have a margin of error of plus or minus ten beats per minute. A twenty-year-old would have a predicted maximum heart rate of 197 beats per minute, plus or minus ten. This means that all normal twenty-year-olds would have maximum heart rates somewhere between 187 and 207 beats per minute.

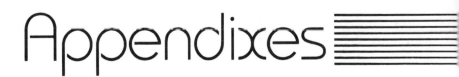

Appendixes

# Appendix 2—Levels of Body Fat (Men)

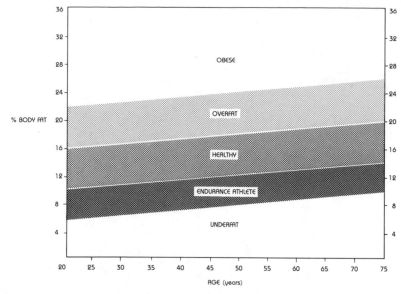

## Levels of Body Fat (Women)

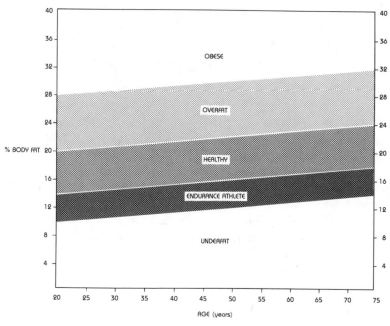

# Appendix 3—Interval Training

| QUANTITY | | | INTERVAL TYPE | | INTENSITY | | |
|---|---|---|---|---|---|---|---|
| | | | work | rest | | | |
| 8 repetitions | 10 repetitions | 12 repetitions | 3 min | 1½ min | 70–80% HR Max | 80–90% HR Max | 90–100% HR Max |
| | | | 2 min | 1 min | | | |
| | | | 1 min | 40 sec | | | |
| | | | 3 | 1 | | | |
| | | | 2 | 45 sec | | | |
| | | | 1 | 30 sec | | | |
| | | | 3 | 45 sec | | | |
| | | | 2 | 30 sec | | | |
| | | | 1 | 15 sec | | | |

☐ = EASY    ▦ = MEDIUM    ▥ = HARD

There are three things to consider in interval training: the quantity, or number of repetitions performed; the type of interval, or the ratio of work to rest; and the intensity of the workout, or the percentage of the maximum heart rate at which the exercise is performed.

Each of these factors has been subdivided to provide workouts that are relatively easy, moderately intense, and difficult. Everything in white (including the quantity, type, and intensity) is relatively easy. Dotted is more difficult, and striped is even more difficult. You do not have to select components from the same level, but you can mix them any way you want.

Start your intense training period with workouts that are relatively easy for you. Then progress to increasingly difficult workouts at your own pace. If you can't complete a workout, go back to an easier level. Don't be discouraged if you can't get to a triple striped workout (striped quantity, type, and intensity), because they are extremely difficult.

## Appendix 4—Age-Predicted Maximal Oxygen Consumption for Healthy Men in Ml/kg·min$^{-1}$

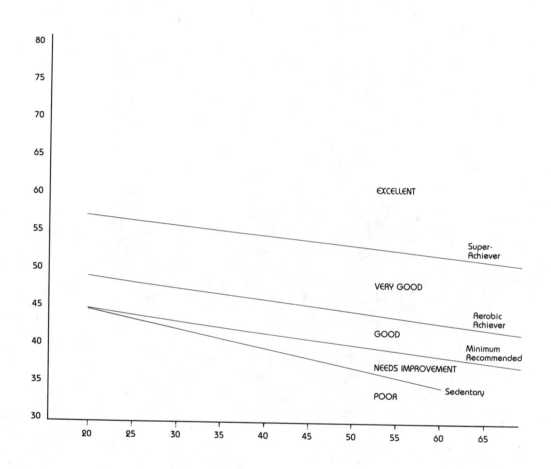

# Age-Predicted Maximal Oxygen Consumption for Healthy Women in Ml/kg·min$^{-1}$

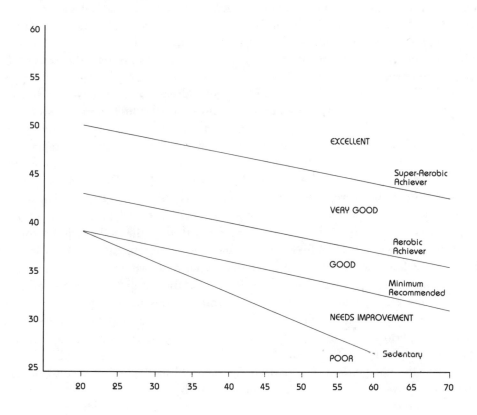

Sedentary—Free from disease but nonexercising

Minimum Recommended—Moderate aerobic activity for approximately twenty minutes, each session approximately three times per week

Aerobic Achiever—Moderate aerobic activity in sessions longer than thirty minutes, five to seven times per week

Super-Aerobic Achiever—Moderate- to high-intensity aerobic activity, approximately sixty minutes per session, five to seven times per week

# Appendix 5—Glycogen- (Carbo-) Loading

Glycogen-loading, which is the correct term for what commonly is called carbo-loading, refers to the method by which the glycogen stores in the muscles can be increased above normal levels. It can improve muscle glycogen levels as much as two times normal levels, and is used by people preparing for endurance events, such as marathons and triathlons. There are several ways to glycogen load, but all begin six to seven days before the event.

The classical method of glycogen-loading can increase the carbohydrate stores in the muscles to up to two times the normal level. In the first three days of the week, derive only 10 to 15 percent of your calories from carbohydrate sources, 35 to 40 percent from protein, and 50 percent from fat. On the first day of the regimen, work out for ninety minutes to two hours at a moderate intensity, so that the muscle glycogen stores in your body become as depleted as possible. On the second and third days, do light exercise of approximately thirty minutes' duration. On days four through seven, switch to a diet composed of 75 percent carbohydrates, 10 percent protein, and 10–15 percent fat. By the fourth day, the carbohydrate stores in the muscles will be virtually depleted, and the change to high carbohydrates will allow the body to store more glycogen than it normally would. Some authorities advise complete rest during these last days prior to the competition, while others (including myself) recommend light exercise until the day before the event.

Some coaches feel that an exhaustive exercise session six days before competition may impede performance in the event itself. Others believe that athletes are likely to feel tired, listless, and psychologically disadvantageous from eating a high-fat diet so near the competition. I have used the classical method of glycogen-loading many times, however, and never had a problem with it.

If you are concerned about either problem, vary the method by eliminating the first exercise session. Perform only light exercise daily throughout the week. While this will be less effective than the first strategy, it can produce loading of glycogen stores to about 60 percent greater than normal.

Switching from a normal diet directly to a high-carbohydrate, low-fat diet in the week before competition can also help. Because you control the intake of fats, you won't feel listless, can increase glycogen stores about 20 percent, and still enhance your performance.

# Appendix 6—The Effects of Hydration on Performance

Proper hydration is important in all sporting endeavors, but it can be and often is the limiting factor in endurance activities. In some sports, the fluid losses are tremendous—a one hundred sixty-pound man can easily lose over two liters of fluid per hour through sweating and breathing out water vapor from the lungs. Some cross-country skiers, in fact, have recorded losses of five liters per hour. Think about five quarts of milk in your refrigerator and the staggering quantity of this amount will become apparent.

When fluid losses are not replaced, the body's core temperature rises and performance suffers. You don't have to lose five liters, either. Losses of only 3 percent of your body weight will negatively affect performance. When these losses get to be about 7–8 percent of your body weight, the potential for danger increases dramatically because major organ damage, particularly of the kidneys, can occur. Many, if not most, competitors in marathons and triathlons finish their events with weight losses in the 4–6 percent range, so this is not an academic or only occasional problem.

Hydration is complicated by the fact that the stomach can absorb only a finite amount of fluid in a given amount of time. A one hundred sixty-pound man, for example, can absorb only a little over one liter of fluid per hour, regardless of how much fluid he has lost. You can drink much more than that one liter, but the excess will not be absorbed. The only way to guarantee steady performance is to replace the fluid regularly throughout the athletic activity.

In events that last less than two-and-a-half hours, water is the only replenishment needed. If, like most people, you take longer to finish your marathon, cross-country ski race, triathlon, or long bike tour, include a small amount of calories in the fluid intake.

Monitor the caloric content of the fluid carefully, however, because any caloric concentration of over 4 percent (4 percent sugar, 96 percent water) substantially increases the time it takes the stomach to empty. The average soft drink is about a 10-percent sugar solution, and most of the so-called sport drinks are in the 6–7½ percent range. One of the country's most eminent physiologists, Dave Costill, has published data indicating that sugar solutions of 2½ percent are best for endurance events lasting longer than two hours. My own research with triathletes exercising continuously for eight hours (longer than in any other published study) showed that drinking a 4-percent carbohydrate solution maintains good hydration as well as normal blood sugar.

Whenever fluid replacement is critical, such as in hot-weather tennis, long-distance running, or cross-country skiing, replenish fluids regularly and a little at a time. To maintain safe hydration levels, a one hundred sixty-pound man should drink approximately a cup of fluid every fifteen minutes. Adjust the exact amount to your own weight, but maintain the fifteen-minute schedule.

To control the rate of emptying in the stomach in triathlons and other sports, consume only fluids. In the study I did, eight elite triathletes ate a variety of solid foods for the eight-hour exercise session (five hours of cycling and three hours of running). Then, two weeks later, they did the same exercise, consuming only a dilute (4-percent) sugar solution during the workout. In the first exercise session, they averaged a 5-percent loss of their body weight. In the second session, their weight loss was under 3 percent, or well within safe limits. In addition, their performance times and their subjective appraisal of their efforts were much better during the fluid-only day.

For day-long skiing, bicycle touring, tennis, and other endurance activities where there is a sustained and fairly intense effort, you thus will do better not by eating solid food but with smaller fluid meals, such as soups, juice, and cocoa. This is not good news to the many skiers who understandably feel that a leisurely midday stop at a quaint hillside restaurant is half the fun of skiing, but it is optimal sports nutrition.

## Books

Astrand, P. O., and Rodahl, K. *Textbook of Work Physiology* (2d ed.). New York: McGraw-Hill Publishing Co., 1977.

Betts, J. M., and Eichelberger, M., eds. *Clinics in Sports Medicine—Pediatric and Adolescent Sports Medicine*. Philadelphia: W. B. Saunders Co., 1982.

Cohen, L. S., Mock, M. B. and Ringquist, I. *Physical Conditioning and Cardiovascular Rehabilitation*. New York: John Wiley & Sons, 1981.

Ficat, R. P., and Hungerford, D. S. *Disorders of the Patello-Femoral Joint*. Baltimore: Williams & Wilkins, 1977.

Frankel, V. H., and Nordin, M. *Biomechanics of the Skeletal System*. Philadelphia: Lea & Febiger, 1980.

Haskell, W., Scala, J., and Whittam, J., eds. *Nutrition and Athletic Performance*. Palo Alto, Calif.: Bull Publishing Co., 1982.

Heath, D., and Williams, D. R. *Man at High Altitude*. New York: Churchill Livingstone, 1981.

Hutton, R. S., and Miller, D. I., eds. *Exercise and Sports Sciences Reviews*. Vol. 8, 1980. Philadelphia: The Franklin Institute Press, 1981.

Jobe, P. W., ed. *Clinics in Sports Medicine—Injuries to the Shoulder in the Athlete*. Philadelphia: W. B. Saunders Co., 1983.

Katz, M., and Stiehm, E. R. *Comprehensive Manuals in Pediatrics—Pediatric Sports Medicine for the Practitioner*. New York: Springer-Verlag, 1983.

O'Donaghue, D. H. *Treatment of Injuries to Athletes*. Philadelphia: W. B. Saunders Co., 1976.

Sammarco, G. J., ed. *Clinics in Sports Medicine—Injuries to Dancers*. Philadelphia: W. B. Saunders Co., 1984.

Sheon, R. P., Moskowitz, R. W., and Goldberg, V. M. *Soft Tissue Rheumatic Pain: Recognition, Management, Prevention*. Philadelphia: Lea & Febiger, 1982.

Stanton-Hicks, M., and Boas, R. A., eds. *Chronic Low Back Pain*. New York: Raven Press, 1982.

Strauss, R. H. *Sportsmedicine*. Philadelphia: W. B. Saunders, 1984.

Torg, J. S., ed. *Clinics in Sports Medicine—Ankle and Foot Problems in the Athlete*. Philadelphia: W. B. Saunders Co., 1982.

Walsh, W. M., ed. *Clinics in Sports Medicine—the Athletic Woman*. Philadelphia: W. B. Saunders Co., 1984.

# Bibliography

Zarins, B., ed. *Clinics in Sports Medicine—Olympic Sports Medicine.* Philadelphia: W. B. Saunders Co., 1983.

## Articles

Abraham, W. M. "Factors in Delayed Muscle Soreness." *Med. Sci. Sports*, Vol. 9, Spring 1977.

Armstrong, R. B., Garshnek, V., Schwane, J. A. "Muscle Inflammation: Response to Eccentric Exercise, Abstracted," *Med. Sci. Sports Exerc.*, Vol. 12, No. 2, 1980.

Armstrong, R. B., Ogilvie, R. W., Schwane, J. A. "Eccentric Exercise-Induced Injury to Rat Skeletal Muscle." *J. Appl. Physiol.*, Vol. 54, Jan. 1983.

Bergstrom, J., Hermansen, L., Hultman, E., et.al. "Diet, Muscle Glycogen, and Physical Performance." *Acta Physiol. Scand.*, Vol. 71, Oct.–Nov. 1967.

Bruce, R. A. "Exercise, Functional Aerobic Capacity, and Aging—Another Viewpoint." *Med. Sci. Sports Exer.*, Vol. 16, No. 1, 1984.

Buchbinder, M. R., Napora, N. J., Biggs, E. W. "The Relationship of Abnormal Pronation to Chondramalacia of the Patella in Distance Runners." *J. Am. Podiatry Assoc.*, Vol. 69, No. 2, 1979.

Caldwell, F. "Bindings: A Criticial Role in Downhill Ski Safety." *Phy. Sportsmed.*, Vol. 12, No. 1, Jan. 1984.

Caldwell, F. "Epidemiology in Sports Medicine Overview: Epidemiologists Take Their Place on the Sports Medicine Team." *Phy. Sportmed*, Vol. 13, No. 3, Mar. 1985.

Costill, D. L., Thomason, H., and Roberts, E. "Fractional Utilization of the Aerobic Capacity During Distance Running." *Med. Sci. Sports*, Vol. 5, Winter 1973.

Costill, D. L. "Metabolic Responses During Distance Running." *J. Appl. Physiol.*, Vol. 28, Mar. 1970.

Costill, D. L. "Physiology of Marathon Running." *JAMA*, Vol. 221, Aug. 28, 1972.

Crews, D. "A Physiological Profile of Ladies Professional Golf Association Tour Players." *Phys. Sportsmed*, Vol. 12, No. 5, May 1984.

Davis, J. A., Vodak, P., Wilmore, J. H., et.al. "Anaerobic Threshold and Maximal Aerobic Power for Three Modes of Exercise." *J. Appl. Physiol.*, Vol. 441, Oct. 1976.

Ellsworth, N. M., Hewitt, B. F., Haskell, W. L. "Nutrient Intake of Elite Male and Female Nordic Skiers." *Phys. Sportsmed*, Vol. 13, No. 2, Feb. 1985.

Farrell, P. A., Wilmore, J. H., Coyle, E. F., et. al. "Plasma Lactate Accumulation and Distance Running Performance." *Med. Sci. Sports*, Vol. 2, Winter 1979.

Feigley, D. A. "Psychological Burnout in High-Level Athletes." *Phys. Sportsmed.*, Vol. 12, No. 10, Oct. 1984.

Forsythe, K. "Force-Velocity Relationship in Runners." *Med. Sci. Sports Exercise*, Vol. 15, No. 3, 1983.

Francis, L. L., Francis, P. R., Welshons-Smith, K. "Aerobic Dance Injuries: A Survey of Instructors," *Phys. Sportsmed.*, Vol. 13, No. 2, Feb. 1985.

Frederick, E. C. "Synthesis, Experimentation, and the Biomechanics of Economical Movement." *Med. Sci. Sports Exer.*, Vol. 17, No. 1, 1985.

Friedman, D. B., Ramo, B. W., Gray, G. J. "Tennis and Cardiovascular Fitness." *Phys. Sportsmed.*, Vol. 12, No. 7, July 1984.

Greenleaf, J. E. "Physiology of Fluid and Electrolyte Responses During Inactivity: Water Immersion and Bed Rest." *Med. Sci. Sports Exer.*, Vol. 16, No. 1, 1984.

Gwinup, G. "Effect of Exercise Alone on the Weight of Obese Women." *Arch. Int. Med.*, Vol. 135, May 1975.

Hagerman, F. C., Hikida, R. S., Staron, R. S., et al. "Muscle Damage in Marathon Runners," *Phys. Sportsmed.*, Vol. 12, No. 11, Nov. 1984.

Johnson, R. W., and Morgan, W. P. "Personality Characteristics of College Athletes in Different Sports." *Scand. J. Sports Sci.*, Vol. 3, 1981.

Jones, N. "Dyspnea in Exercise." *Med. Sci. Sports Exer.*, Vol. 16, No. 1, 1984.

Keesey, R. "A Set-Point Analysis of the Regulation of Body Weight." In *Obesity*, by A. J. Stunkard. Philadelphia: W. B. Saunders, 1980.

Komi, P. V., and Busbirk, E. R., "The Effect of Eccentric and Concentric Muscle Activity on Tension and Electrical Activity of Human Muscle." *Ergonomics*, Vol. 15, July 1972.

Komi, P. V. "Biomechanics and Neuromuscular Performance." *Med. Sci. Sports Exer.*, Vol. 16, No. 1, 1984.

LaPorte, R. E., Adams, L. L., Savage, D. D., et al. "The Spectrum of Physical Activity, Cardiovascular Disease and Health: An Epidemiologic Perspective." *Am. J. Epidemiol.*, Vol. 120, Oct. 1984.

LaPorte, R. E., and Blair, S. N. "Physical Activity or Cardiovascular Fitness: Which Is More Important For Health? A Pro and Con." *Phys. Sportsmed.*, Vol. 13, No. 3, Mar. 1985.

Legwold, G. "Does Aerobic Dance Offer More Fun Than Fitness?" *Phys. Sportsmed.*, Vol. 10, Sept. 1982.

Leon, A. S., Blackburn, H. "The Relationship of Physical Activity to Coronary Heart Disease and Life Expectancy." *Ann. NY Acad. Sci.*, Vol. 301, 1977.

Leon, A. S., Conrad, J., Hunninghake, D. B., et al. "Effects of a Vigorous Walking Program on Body Composition, and Carbohydrate and Lipid Metabolism of Obese Young Men." *Am. J. Clin. Nutr.*, vol. 32, Sept. 1979.

Lewis, S., Haskell, W. L., Wood, P. D., et al. "Effects of Physical Activity on Weight Reduction in Obese Middle Aged Women." *Am. J. Clin. Nutr.*, Vol. 29, Feb. 1976.

Lindenberg, G. "Illiotibial Band Friction Syndrome in Runners." *Phys. Sportsmed.*, Vol. 12, No. 5, May 1984.

Lohman, T. G., Pollock, M. L., Slaughter, M. H., Brandon, L. J., et al. "Methodological Factors and the Prediction of Body Fat in Female Athletes." *Med. Sci. Sports Exer.*, Vol. 16, No. 1, 1984.

Loucks, A. B., and Horvath, S. B. "Athletic Amenorrhea: A Review." *Med. Sci. Sports Exer.*, Vol. 17, No. 1, 1985.

Maron, M. B., Horvath, S. M. "The Marathon: A History and Review of the Literature." *Med. Sci. Sports*, Vol. 10, Summer 1978.

Martin, B. J., Chen, H., and Kolka, M. A. "Anaerobic Metabolism of the Respiratory Muscles During Exercise." *Med. Sci. Sports Exer.*, Vol. 16, No. 1, 1984.

Martin, B. J., and Chen, H. "Sleep Loss and the Sympathoadrenal Response to Exercise." *Med. Sci. Sports Exer.*, Vol. 16, No. 1, 1984.

Morgan, W. P. "Affective Beneficence of Vigorous Physical Activity." *Med. Sci. Sports Exer.*, Vol. 17, No. 1, 1985.

Morgan, W. P. "Selected Psychological Considerations in Sports." *Res. Q. Am. Assoc. Health Phys. Educ.*, Vol. 45, Dec. 1974.

Morgan, W. P., and Pollock, M. L. "Psychological Characteristics of the Elite Distance Runner." *Ann. NY Acad. Sci.*, Vol. 301, Oct. 1977.

Morgans, L. F., Scovil, J. A., and Bass, K. M. "A Comparison of Heart Rate Responses During Singles and Doubles Competition in Racquetball." *Phys. Sportsmed.*, Vol. 12, No. 11, Nov. 1984.

Nagle, F. G., Morgan, W. P., and Hellickson, R. O., et al. "Spotting Success Traits in Olympic Contenders." *Phys. Sportsmed.*, Vol. 3, 1975.

Oyster, N., Morton, M., and Linnell, S. "Physical Activity and Osteoporosis in Post-Menopausal Women." *Med. Sci. Sports Exer.*, Vol. 16, No. 1, 1984.

Paffenbarger, R. S., Hyde, R. T., Wing, A. L., et al. "A Natural History of Athletics and Cardiovascular Health." *JAMA*, Vol. 252, July 27, 1984.

Parr, R. B. "Iron Deficiency in Female Athletes." *Phys. Sporstmed.*, Vol. 12, No. 4, Apr. 1984.

Pate, R. R. "Sports Anemia: A Review of the Current Research Literature." *Phys. Sportsmed.*, Vol. 11, No. 2, Feb. 1983.

Puranen, J. "The Medial Tibial Syndrome: Exercise Ischemia in the Medial Fascial Compartment of the Leg." *J. Bone Joint Surg.*, Vol. 56B, Nov. 1984.

Rhodes, E. C. "Predicted Marathon Time From Anaerobic Threshold Measurements." *Phys. Sportsmed.*, Vol. 12, No. 1, Jan. 1984.

Richie, D. H., Kelso, S. F. and Bellucci, P. A. "Aerobic Dance Injuries: A Retrospective Study of Instructors and Participants," *Phys. Sportsmed.*, Vol. 13, No. 2, Feb. 1985.

Rogers, C. C., ed. "The Los Angeles Olympic Games: Effects of Pollution Unclear." *Phys. Sports Med.*, Vol. 12, No. 2, May 1984.

Schwane, J. A., Johnson, S. R., Vandenakker, C. B., et al. "Delaying-Onset Muscular Soreness and Plasma CPK and LDH Activities After Downhill Running." *Med. Sci. Sports Exer.*, Vol. 15, No. 1, 1983.

Siegel, A. J., Hennekens, C. H., Solomon, H. S., et al. "Exercise-Related Hematuria." *JAMA*, Vol. 241, Jan. 26, 1979.

Sinning, W. E., Dolny, D. G., Little, R. D., et al. "Validity of 'Generalized' Equations for Body Composition Analysis in Male Athletes." *Med. Sci. Sports Exer.*, Vol. 17, No. 1, 1985.

Sjodin, B., and Jacobs, I. "Onset of Blood Lactate Accumulation and Marathon Running Performance," *Int. J. Sports Med. II*, Vol. 1, 1981.

Smith, M. H. "Altitude Training: Who Benefits?" *Phys. Sportsmed.*, Vol. 12, No. 4, Apr. 1984.

Standish, W. D. "Overuse Injuries in Athletes: A Perspective." *Med. Sci. Sports Exer.*, Vol. 16, Jan. 1984.

Sullivan, S. N., Champion, M. D., Christofides, N. D., et al. "Gastrointestinal Regulatory Peptide Responses in Long-Distance Runners." *Phys. Sportsmed.*, Vol. 12, No. 7, July 1984.

Sutton, J. R. "Endorphins in Exercise." *Med. Sci. Sports Exer.*, Vol. 17, No. 1, 1985.

Tesch, P. "Muscle Fatigue in Man." *Acta Physiologica Scand.*, Suppl. 480, 1980.

Upton, S. G., Hagan, R. D., Lease, B., et al. "Comparative Physiological Profiles Among Young and Middle-Aged Female Distance Runners." *Med. Sci. Sports Exer.*, Vol. 16, No. 1, 1984.

Vetter, W. L., Helfet, D. L., Spear, K., et al. "Aerobic Dance Injuries." *Phys. Sportsmed.*, Vol. 13, No. 2, Feb. 1985.

Warren, B. L. "Anatomical Factors Associated with Predicting Plantar Fasciitis in Long-Distance Runners." *Med. Sci. Sports Exer.*, Vol. 16, No. 1, 1984.

Washington, E. L. "Musculoskeletal Injuries in Theatrical Dancers: Site, Frequency and Severity." *Am. J. Sportsmed.*, Vol. 6, Mar.–Apr. 1978.

Wasserman, K., and Whipp, B. G., "Exercise Physiology in Health and Disease." *Am. Rev. Respir. Dis.*, Aug. 1975.

Wasserman, K., Whipp, B. G., Koyal, S. N., et al. "Anaerobic Threshold and Respiratory Gas Exchange During Exercise." *J. Appl. Physiol.*, Vol. 35, Aug. 1973.

Weltman, A., Malter, S., and Stanford, B. "Caloric Restriction and/or Mild Exercise: Effects on Serum Lipids and Body Composition." *Am. J. Clin. Nutr.*, Vol. 33, May 1980.

Winder, W. W. "Control of Hepatic Glucose Production During Exercise." *Med. Sci. Sports Exer.*, Vol. 17, No. 1, 1985.

Woo, R., Garrow, J., and Pi-Sunger, F. "Effect of Exercise on Spontaneous Calorie Intake in Obesity Abstracted." *Clin. Res.*, Vol. 29, Apr. 1981.

Wood, P. D., Haskell, W. L., Terry, R. B., et al. "Effects of a Two-Year Running Program on Plasma Lipoproteins, Body Fat, and Dietary Intake in Initially Sedentary Men." *Med. Sci. Sports Exer.*, Vol. 14, 1982.